Healing the Womb

A Journey to Wellness and Wholeness

Carol Lynne Smith

HEALING THE WOMB: A JOURNEY TO WELLNESS AND WHOLENESS
CAROL LYNNE SMITH

Scripture quotations are taken from THE HOLY BIBLE, NEW INTERNATIONAL VERSION®, NIV®

Published by Pecan Tree Publishing
April 2019
Hollywood, FL
www.pecantreebooks.com

978-1-7328311-0-0 Paperback
978-1-7328311-1-7 Ebook
Library of Congress Control Number: 2018959197

Cover and Interior Design by: www.peacockdesign.pro
Cover Photo by: Michael Anthony Clark

Contents

Pecan Tree Publishing
www.pecantreebooks.com
Hollywood, FL

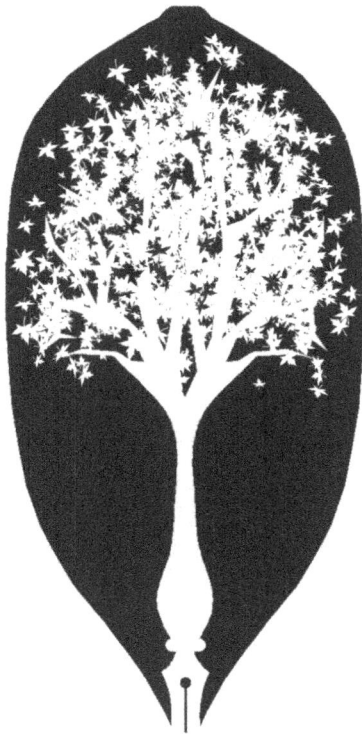

New Voices | New Styles | New Vision –
Creating a New Legacy of Dynamic Authors and Titles

CAROL'S PASSION TOUCHES LIVES

---— ✳ —---

My dear Carol has been a huge part of my journey since I moved to Fort Lauderdale in 2010.

I've had the pleasure of being able to be myself around her without judgement. She has helped me with major life issues and minor day-to-day things that - realistically - I should be able to tackle myself yet I know she's always a phone call away and I'm forever thankful for that. This world is a much better place for knowing I can call Carol Lynne Smith, my friend and my mentor.

Shaunette H.

Where do I start? I knew my life called for my goals to be out of the ordinary. The weight loss, financial gain, and traveling more was not going to cut it for me. I wanted more out of life; but couldn't pinpoint what I wanted. I started to write down my voids: passion in my marriage, disconnection from my children, planning for the future and preparing for the unexpected; time with family to show my appreciation.

I decided to contact Carol Lynne; not really thinking that I could use her assistance, but just to ask some questions about meditation and bringing positivity in my life. I noticed something spectacular had happened in Carol's life. I admire the positivity that radiates from her;

and how she can motivate not only me - but others. I said, "that is the type of energy I need to surround myself with."

Carol blew my mind with her knowledge and wisdom. Carol recommended that I do a Chakra reading to guide me with my goals. I thought that sounded spooky, although I was not practicing or connected to anything spiritually at that time. I just didn't want to take part in anything that would push me further away from God. With that said, Carol recommended that I do some research on the Chakra reading and let me know if I would like to meet. After research, we met; and she read my chakras. I immediately felt the presence of God speak to me, "I have never left your side, no matter how many times you doubted me." The feeling of healing is priceless.

At that very moment, I knew my void was my relationship with God. The space that I am in now – is like I can't get enough of God! I have reconnected with my daughter who had been distant from me. The passion is back in my marriage. My son, who I have struggled with emotionally and thought was suffering from depression, is now the son I could never dream of and more! When it comes to my business, I have learned to work smarter and not harder; while putting God first in everything that I do. I am still a work in progress, however I am proud to say I am well on my way. Carol, thank you so much, and I pray that God continues to guide you and give you the strength to heal others!

Shonae S.

I met Carol when we were working for the same company. I would always pay attention to her talking about all the natural methods she uses - sage, crystals etc. One day we had a conversation about me being a first-time mom and learning how not to be that overly fearful, over-protective parent to my son. We talked about her grounding bowl and its benefits, and she explained the difference in each of the crystals she uses. She created a grounding bowl for me; in fact, a yellow grounding bowl with a couple of things in it like dried flowers, soil, sand and other things from the earth.

That night she called me and explained all the benefits and meaning of each object or material in it. I wasn't sure it would work but I followed all of Carol's instructions. I created a little space for myself to start meditating (something I never was into). The next night I sat and meditated with the grounding bowl. I wanted to find peace about doing the best job possible as a new mom; and be comforted knowing that my son is okay. I meditated and took it all in the sand from the beach for the relaxation, the soil from her dad's yard that meant so much to her. Once I was done meditating, there was a feeling that could not be explained in writing or spoken words. It was an experience that I never knew was possible.

I now meditate every single night and can now sleep the whole night (like my son); and not wake up frantic about whether he is breathing, too hot, too cold, protected, okay. Taking in all the parental advice from everywhere, had become overwhelming and honestly, I didn't think I would find that inner peace. Through the grounding bowl, using sage, and crystals, I was able to successfully let all that go. Carol showed me how to find that peace that seemed so far away.

Alex D.

Healing the Womb

A Journey to Wellness and Wholeness

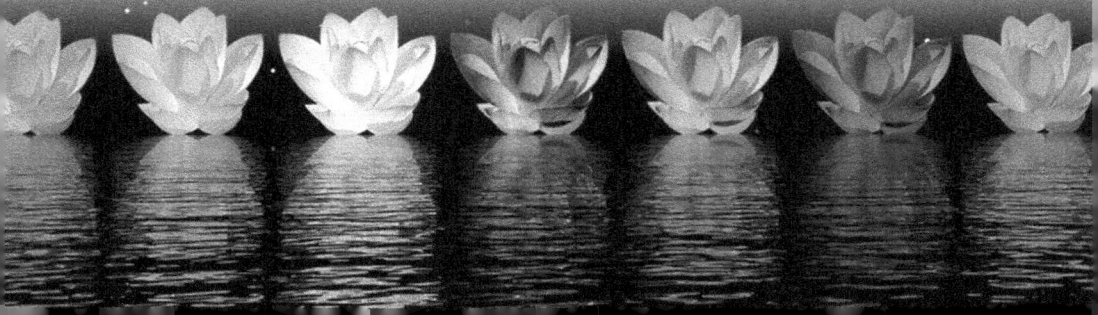

FOREWORD

---*---

It was the most God-awful pain I had ever experienced. I was convinced there was a legion of corrupt little demons living in my uterus who would randomly conduct stabbing parties therein. The only thing more vicious than that was the repeated birthing of clots. I would find myself in a birthing squat repeatedly at work, hid away in bathrooms or behind locked doors. In my mind, that position offered some relief. It beckoned the pain to exit. Fibroid tumors were consuming me internally; externally their ravenous ways were beginning to show.

I was in the lounge at work one morning, fixing a cup of tea, when Kim walked in. She stopped abruptly, looked at me in a concerned fashion and asked if I was alright. I told her I was in a little pain, but fine otherwise, then inquired about her question. She said, "I could be wrong, but I don't think your skin should be pink. You do know you are pink, right?"

I did not know I was pink. She thought we should call for emergency personnel. I protested and drove myself to the emergency room, where I was immediately admitted and prepped for a blood transfusion. The nurse indicated that I was in crisis. I didn't feel any differently. I didn't feel crisis in my body. I had been in pain and critically anemic for so long that it had become my new normal. My new normal – had it not been for divine intervention through Kim – would have left me dead that day.

A few weeks later, I shifted into another new normal. I was a woman without her physical womb. I did not feel less than a woman; yet I was keenly aware that something in the center of my body was missing. It was more than physical. Whatever it was, for weeks I was a hot crying mess. My son would drop a toy – I would cry. My son would get hungry – I would cry. My nephew would ask a question – I would cry. Finally, the 12-year old nephew took charge of the three-year old son and the house. He couldn't figure out why I was crying; but he did what he could to make it stop. That included calling a relative who demanded to know what the crying was about. Was I in menopause? Was I in pain? I had no words to explain it.

Finally, what I know now was a period of mourning for natural children I would not birth (my son is adopted); for accepting life fleeing my body without battle; for the hollowness in my soul and spirit revealed through a major physical removal of a part of me – ended.

There were other parts of me that were awakened powerfully during that time. I was awakened as an empath. I was awakened as a prophetic dreamer. I was awakened - reawakened – to the depth of which I felt people's pains and stories. This time, I had to find a way to release what I would take in before. I had taken it all in and held it in my womb like a concerned mother – even things that were never mine to take in. I poured into scripts, short fiction, poetry and whatever literary muse was on the menu for the day. I also began a battle with depression and anxiety. This battle rages whenever the junk is overwhelming and fights to rest some place within me again. I stubbornly resist.

I did not know my womb could be healed. By the time I had a hysterectomy; I had already undergone a myomectomy. My focus was on getting rid of the pain, never healing the diseased womb or the spiritual womb that remained. As I watched Carol move through her procedure and then the post-surgery mending; I also noticed her infusion of other modalities to welcome healing. It was refreshing to me. It ignited something in me, and I began to face some things generationally, spiritually and emotionally that my womb had been trying to tell me for years.

I still have work to do on my womb healing journey. She (my womb) still cries like a little girl compassionately wanting someone to listen to her. I see, vividly, who she will be when her healing is complete. This book is my personal invitation to sit down for tea with the three of us and become a woman who is an increasing force to be reckoned with. That is what I hope this prescription for healing will be for you as well – an invitation to live in the power that longs to awaken in you.

E. Claudette Freeman

BEYOND THE CLIFF

I stood there
on that cliff –
determined that I would jump!
Too many vacated vows
and empty promises
Far too many "I don't love you anymore"
words spoken
Blackened eyes,
broken skin,
concealed bruises
Empty smiles
underneath vacant eyes.

So, there I stood –
on that cliff
It was then that I noticed it.

There was more beyond the cliff –
a meadow full
of beautiful yellow flowers
Lush green mountains
Flowing bodies of water
The Horizon.

There was so much more beyond the cliff.
There is always so much more beyond the cliff.

INTO THE WOODS

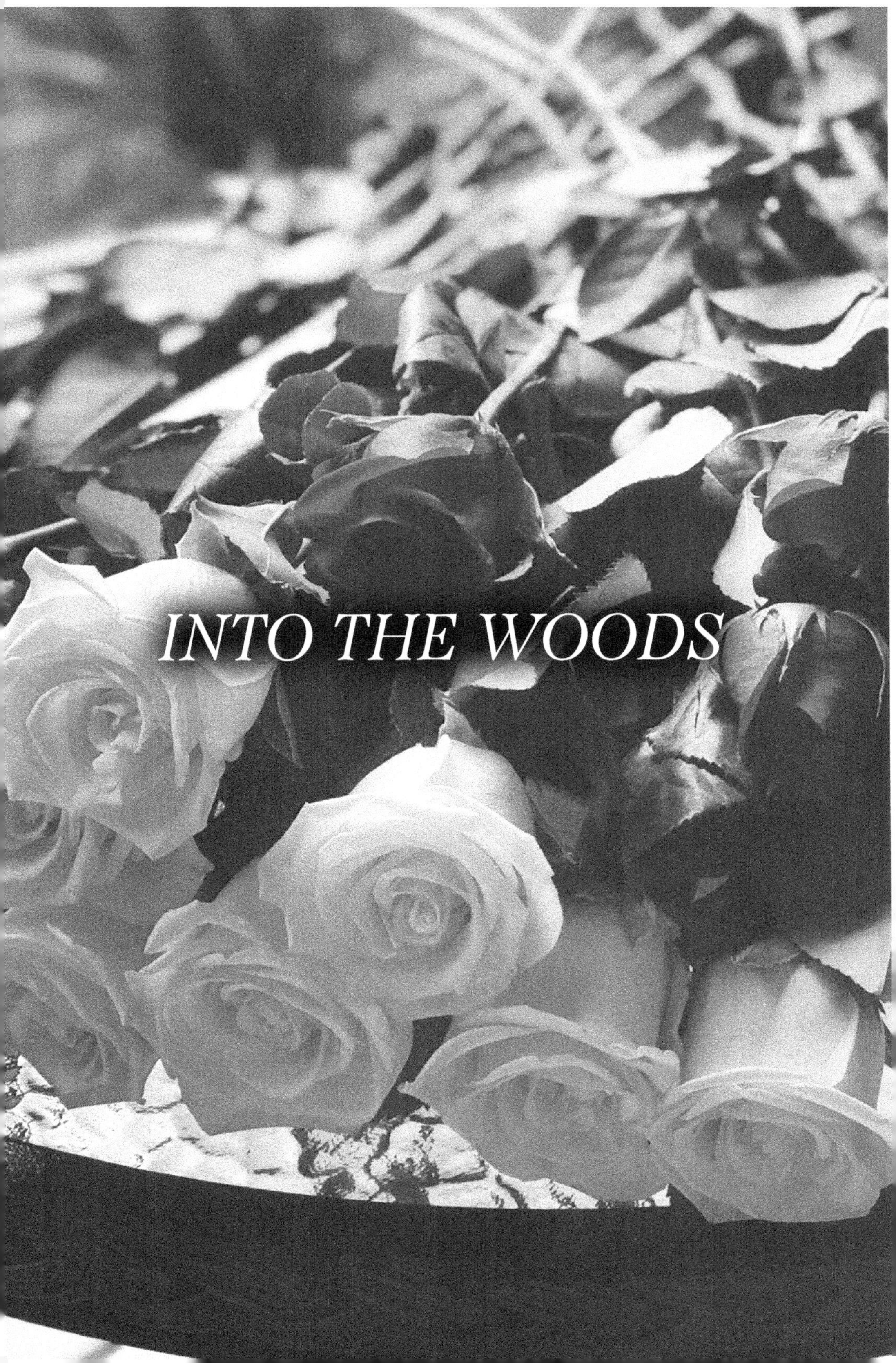

An Introduction

———————✳———————

It was 1996, during a routine yearly exam, that I heard the word "fibroid" for the first time. I was told that it was about the size of a quarter and there was no need to be concerned. Although it presented no real cause for concern at the time, I was never told what could happen if the issue was not monitored or addressed. Twenty years later, I laid on a gurney in an emergency room, being told I had six - to eight - hours to live.

What happened over that 20-year period was years of self-neglect in so many areas of my life, and it was culminating on a day that usually carried so much joy for me - Christmas. What started as a singular fibroid tumor in 1996 had multiplied to more than 70 tumors, with some as large as a grapefruit. I was not ignorant to the tumors, I knew they were there. My uterus had grown to the size of a woman in her fifth month of pregnancy. My moon (menstrual) cycles were unbearable, and there were times when the pain made me feel like I was dying. I would talk myself through those unbearable moments and remind myself that the pain was temporary; until it wasn't.

On that day, after hours of seeing me extremely sick and growing sicker by the hour, my daughter called for help. My cousin came to take me to the hospital, and that visit to the emergency room saved my life.

The fibroid tumors had been feasting on my blood for years, worsening over that last year. On that day, they were trying to take the little blood I had left.

I was severely anemic, and my blood level was dropping rapidly. Without proper treatment at the hospital, I would have been dead within a few hours.

I recall my children getting sick with everything from; strep throat, croup cough, dog bites to bee stings. Every time one of them got ill, I wasted no time getting them treated. But when it came time to care for myself, I was neglectful. It wasn't just my physical health; there were so many areas of my life where I had managed to put the needs of others above my own; and there I was being told I was gravely ill because of it.

I spent a few days in the hospital getting lifesaving treatments. One month after my first hospital stay, I was back in the hospital, but this time it was to have my physical womb surgically removed. My uterus was beyond repair, and because I had waited so long, a full hysterectomy was my only choice.

My life has been transformed since that Christmas Day, and the journey I now find myself on has been incredible. I am grateful for the extraordinary changes that have taken place in the time since then, but I am filled with a lot of regret.

How much time did I lose by neglecting myself for so long? What amazing experiences did I miss out on because I was so sick? How much damage have I done to my body due to 20 years of neglect?

I cannot get those years back, but here I am with this amazing opportunity to make the absolute most out of the rest of the years that remain. I needed to choose a healthier lifestyle.

Chapter 1

---※---

Why Fibroids?

The cause of uterine fibroids is still a mystery, and without a real clue as to the cause, prevention is non-existent currently. There is varied speculation as to what causes the occurrences of fibroids, but it boils down to an educated guess. What is known is that uterine fibroids occur more often in African-American women than in White women; and it is also believed that having a green diet aids in protecting women from developing this condition.

Without having any concrete knowledge as to the physical or genetic cause of fibroids, many cite emotional causes.

I first started dealing with painful abdominal issues early in my life, probably when I was about thirteen years old. I was dealing with a lot of emotional stress, and although my parents were available, I felt isolated in my pain. I internalized my emotional pain while displaying a smile. I was suffering, but no one knew it. I thought I was being brave, but I was young, naive and in desperate need of help. Help I did not get because my smile and my laughter hid my pain. I swallowed it.

I spent the next 33 years swallowing my pain and showcasing my smile. Not even the people closest to me knew the amount of pain I was in; though they were aware of what I was experiencing. Many were aware that I was having marital issues. Some were aware that my relationships were ending against my will or desire; but so many were unaware of my emotional suffering.

I kept smiling! I kept swallowing!

Abusive relationship; GULP! End of relationship; GULP! Loss of job; GULP! Loss of income; GULP! Issues with my children; GULP! Rape; GULP! My grandmother robbed and murdered; GULP! Losing my dad; GULP! My mother diagnosed with dementia; GULP! Every situation I endured; GULP! I swallowed it all.

I thought I was being brave, but what I was actually doing was turning my body into a toxic wasteland, and I truly believe that by doing so, I turned my womb; the very place where everything is generated; into a nurturing space for fibroids to develop, exist and flourish.

Culturally, women are taught that we can be weak, and we can rely on our men to care for us. That rule does not always translate to every group of women. African-American women, for example are taught that we must be strong. In a world where African-American men are disproportionately imprisoned for minor offenses; unemployed or underemployed; we have had to take on the roles of heads of household and in some cases, we need to act as both mother and father to our children. It was not very long ago when Black women were whipped and raped, and then sent into the fields to work. Internalizing physical and emotional pain seems to be part of our DNA.

Seeking professional help seems to carry so many taboos; I believe it is even more so in my community. I take no pride in this, however it seems that with the help of social media, people are becoming more and more open to expressing their pain, thereby getting help; even if it is from amateur psychologists.

I have long sensed and expressed that many physical ailments began as emotional stressors that were internalized. I was able to tell many people about this, while not taking my own advice; until my health crisis forced me to do so.

Chapter 2

I am Not Okay

The first few days after my surgery, my focus was on my physical healing and comfort. Due to the size of my uterus, I was not a candidate for Laparoscopic surgery, and the traditional surgery left me with a large scar. The focus on my physical healing kept my thoughts occupied; it took me a few weeks to realize that I was not okay. Physically, the surgeons were happy with my recovery, but no one knew just what was going on inside of me. I was not okay.

In the beginning, I chalked those feelings up to the emotional distress of going through a major surgery. The more time that went by, it became more difficult to ignore that I was changing. To my knowledge, none of the women in my family had gone through menopause associated with a hysterectomy, so I did not feel as if I had anyone close enough to me that I could talk with. Historically my sister Lisa was the person I could talk to when I felt I could not talk with anyone else, but she was a few months pregnant, and focused on her own health, and the health of the two little girls growing inside of her. Those weeks after my surgery, I was recovering at home, in my bedroom, and I felt completely isolated from everyone.

Prior to my surgery, all my doctors' appointments were focused on both my surgery, and my post-op healing. There were no conversations about my emotional well-being. There is indeed an emotional response to having your womb removed, but I had no idea what was in store for me.

Chapter 3

―――――※―――――

The Womb

The Womb, or the Uterus, is a cavity or space that resembles a womb in containing and enveloping. Further, according to Merriam-Webster it is a place where *something* is generated. The womb is where life begins and is nurtured for every person. Our womb is our place of creativity and our place of power; the magical place where our soul resides.

Biblically, if a woman could not have children, she was considered -less than- a woman. Women would offer their servants to their husbands to give them children. The same exists within royal families. A woman who can bare heirs is more marriage worthy than one who is barren.

Although I was past the point in my life of having children, the loss of my womb left me with many emotions. I was fearful that I would be disconnected from my womanhood; my femininity.

Was I less of a woman?

Chapter 4

※

But am I a Woman?

It wasn't exceedingly long after my surgery that I began to struggle with issues surrounding my femininity. I read blogs and articles from women who had been thrust into menopause due to a hysterectomy, and all the information carried a similar theme. They all spoke to the link between the womb and womanhood. During this time, I had lost all desire for intimacy, and I felt disconnected from my sexuality. I was afraid that everything that made me feel like a woman was taken away from me on the operating table. I was afraid, and I felt I had no one to talk with.

A few weeks prior to my surgery, I met a woman who several friends told me I needed to meet. Dr. Lanalee Araba Sam. I met her the day I went in to her office to discuss her performing my surgery. She assured me that I was in great hands with her, and she was right of course. The day after my surgery, she came to see me in hospital for a routine, post-op visit. Before she left my room - she told me we would be friends. I thought it was sweet that my surgeon said this to me; I felt she was trying to boost my spirits. It was the day after a major surgery, my hair was a tacky mess and my makeup was a few miles away on my dresser at home. I had not had a shower in about 36 hours, and I was wearing a hideous hospital gown. I appreciated the words she spoke, but I could not imagine there was any weight behind them. I was wrong. Our initial relationship proved beneficial to my physical health, but our friendship would prove beneficial to my emotional well-being.

While I was at home recovering, she began to reach out to me and once I was able to leave home on my own, I would spend time with her at her home on the beach. She would prepare nutritious foods for me, and she offered a library of books for me to read. None of the books she offered were about my physical well-being; she was confident that I was doing well. The books were about my emotional well-being. Our new friendship allowed me the opportunity to open up about where I was emotionally. I felt comfortable chatting with Araba about my feelings because I felt like no one knew me inside and out the way she did (a little surgery humor). Araba began to have conversations with me about things that no one else would have thought to talk with me about. I trusted her, and that allowed me to begin to open up about how I was feeling; lost and disconnected. It was during one of our visits that I was first able to put into words just how "less than" I felt.

Having the ability to verbally express how disconnected I felt, allowed me the opportunity to seek ways to reconnect with myself, my body, my thoughts and my femininity.

Chapter 5

— ✳ —

In the Absence of a Womb

"Even in the absence of the physical Womb, the spiritual womb still exists and needs to be healed." Carol Lynne Smith

I struggled to find resources that addressed the emotional turmoil that I was experiencing as the result of my hysterectomy. That information was not easy to find, and what I discovered was a need to fill that void. My mentor and friend Alison had introduced me to crystals, essential oils and sage. She had spent several years teaching me; through conversation, practice and by her own example just how essential these methods of natural healing were. During my time of need, I looked back on those examples and began to explore their uses for my healing. What I realized was a method of healing through meditations, herbs, crystals, rituals, foods, and ceremonial exercises. An important breakthrough in my healing came when I began to understand the importance of healing the energy within my body. Everything in the Universe is based on vibrational energy. What I soon began to understand was that the womb is the place where our creativity is nurtured and birthed. Even in the absence of a physical womb, there still exist a spiritual womb, and to thrive, that must be healed. To heal, I needed to unblock, align and balance my chi; my life energy.

BEYOND THE CLIFF

Journey- passage or progress

from one stage to another.

Dictionary.com

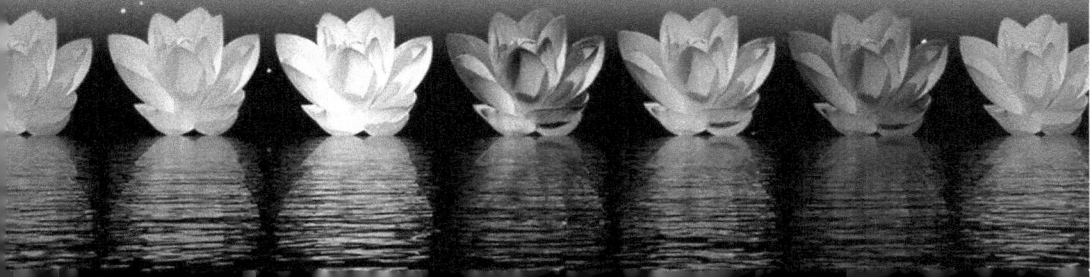

Chapter 6

---✴---

Walking into the Answer

"Don't be confined by conformity – step outside of your comfort zone."
Carol Lynne Smith

The months following my surgery were so difficult. I was desperate to understand everything that was happening inside of me. Intellectually, I understood that change was part of this new journey; but I had no idea how to navigate this new me. My healing research resulted in a bunch of notes in journals, but no clear path. My publisher wanted me to write a book about my healing, but I did not feel healed. Physically, I was much better, but inside of me there was confusion and chaos. I did not know how to tell her that I could not write the book she wanted, at least not then. My publisher and I met for brunch and conversation in order that we might discuss the book she wanted. During our conversation, we were talking about healing crystals (gemstones) and I mentioned that one of my favorite metaphysical shops was nearby, and in fact I told her that I would venture there when we were done meeting. I had no idea how that decision would affect my journey to healing.

Prior to that day, I had reached out to an associate of mine who was an acupuncturist. I knew nothing about the field of acupuncture, but I knew that the roadblocks to my healing were not physical in nature, and I had hoped that an alternative form of healing could tap into the source of my chaos. I walked into the metaphysical store for the purpose of buying a few crystals to wear. My spiritual teacher Alison had convinced me of the healing powers of crystals, and I had been a beneficiary of this manner of healing on several occasions. I wore crystals that had been strung as bracelets and necklaces; when I was feeling anxious or overwhelmed, I would place a crystal named citrine in my bra so that the stone's energy could penetrate my skin. I was a believer, yet there was so much more information I did not have access to, and my ignorance was a roadblock to my healing. I had all the tools needed to heal, but I had no idea how to organize the tools for that purpose.

I walked around the store for a bit, and then I came across the gemstone, chrysocolla. This beautiful blue stone reminded me of my favorite crystal – turquoise, except that it is a more vibrant color of blue. The stone mimics the color of the Caribbean Ocean and it felt like I was holding the entirety of that ocean in the palm of my hand. It was breathtaking!

Vanessa, the woman who worked in the store came over to see if she could help me. I asked her about the healing properties of the stone; balance, new beginnings, change – among other things. Every property it owned resonated with me. Vanessa told me that she had a chrysocolla that she had just wrapped in copper wire and made into a necklace. She gifted it to me. It was beautiful, but that was not the most valuable gift she gave me. When she placed the necklace around my neck, I felt overwhelmed with emotions. She asked me if she could "read my chakras." Intellectually I knew what the chakras were, but I did not have any knowledge of reading them or how that all worked. I happily gave her permission to do so. As she went one-by-one, addressing each area, I could feel my dam bursting. Everything she was saying was true and I would have sworn that she was looking directly inside of me. For months, I walked around smiling at everyone, grateful for my physical health but so isolated and hurt on the inside. Vanessa was the first person who could see me and pinpoint the source of my pain. After the reading was done, she offered me valuable insight into how to heal those areas that had been blocked, and I followed her advice like it was a road map out of a dark tunnel.

I absorbed every piece of information I could about understanding how the chakras work, and how to heal each one. This was a breakthrough to my healing. Suddenly, all the various and scattered notes I had about healing came together and made sense. I had all the medicines I needed to heal my emotional wounds. And thanks to Vanessa, I was able to find the place of my hurt and apply pressure.

WHY DOES ANY OF THIS MATTER?

We are not one-dimensional beings. We are a combination of spirit, soul and body. Womb healing encompasses healing the entire being – spirit, soul and body. Creating an environment where we can heal all aspects of our being, is where we can begin to find wholeness. This journey to wellness and wholeness is a journey of reclaiming the sacred feminine. This is our journey to enlightenment; to proclaiming our power over ourselves, and the environment we seek to create around us. This is our journey to authenticity, renewal, wellness and wholeness. Our healing must be purposeful. We are charged with taking responsibility for it.

Healing the womb means healing from negative relationships, abusive behaviors and allowances; brokenness and negative soul ties. Healing the womb is not just about recovering from a hysterectomy, but also from a harsh monthly cycle, abortion, miscarriage and child birth. Womb healing is about recovering from chronic illness and creating a healthy place where conception can take place. Healing the womb is about preparing a place where something can be birthed from it; whether that be a child, or a creative project.

Healing the womb leads to healing from physical disease and heartache.

Womb healing leads to having healthier relationships with your mother and your own children; it leads to attracting and recognizing your soul's mate. It is about forgiveness, restoration and the releasing of fear. It is about living an outrageously, amazing life that is more beautiful than you could have ever imagined. Healing the womb is about healing the woman. It is all about you!

ALABASTER BOX

There is a biblical story that resonates with me. In the Gospel of Luke, chapter 7, we are introduced to a woman described as a sinner. During this time- for a woman to be called a sinner, it usually meant that she was known for having more than one sexual partner. In this Gospel, we find this woman making her way into the home of someone of great stature in the Jewish community, because she had her mind set on meeting with Jesus.

She came in carrying an expensive bottle of oil that she used for the purpose of anointing Jesus. She became so emotional after meeting Him that she fell at his feet and cried. Using her hair as a towel, she tried to dry her tears off His feet. The homeowner was horrified at this unclean woman touching the Prophet, and even more horrified that Jesus had allowed Himself to be touched by a sinner. After using her hair to dry the tears off the feet of Jesus, the woman kissed His feet and poured the expensive oil on them to anoint Him. As she sat before Him completely humbled, Jesus forgave her for her sins.

I believe this to be a story of womb healing as much as it is about forgiveness.

This is what womb healing is; it is forgiving yourself for whatever you allowed to happen there and forgiving others for the hurt they caused you. To heal, there must be forgiveness. For women of God, this does include petitioning your Creator in prayer and asking for that forgiveness. When we sincerely go before God - confess our hurts, He forgives. That forgiveness is available as often as we need it.

Chapter 7

---※---

Finding Value in the Brokenness, Lest, it be in Vain

On this journey to wellness and wholeness, not every day will feel sunny. There are days where it will be hard to see the sun through the dark clouds. We must trust that she is there; the clouds will part, and we will bask in her rays. We must not lose faith in ourselves, in God or this Universe. There are moments when it will look like we are on the edge of a cliff. The Sun will soon shine, and we will discover that it was not a cliff, it was a breakthrough.

Let us reflect on this. We do not grow based solely on the fact that we experienced something, we grow by reflecting on the experience and absorbing the lesson. We spend so much time complaining about what we are going through - what we are experiencing - that we seldom stop long enough to ask the question, "what is the Universe trying to teach me?"

A visitor to my little Zen place, shared something insightful about these valley engagements. *"When we are in our valley experience, we may also stumble across our human angel. Someone that lifts us up out of our despair and breathes life into our very existence. Someone who gives us reason to feel that we have another chance to fight and that miracles truly do exist. They save us from our own despair. Consider this a true blessing and an extremely huge gain that can be reached when you have hit rock bottom in the valley. I found my angel in human form while I was in the valley."*

We LOVE mountaintop experiences. We value those moments when everything seems to be going our way. We all desire that God blesses us in some major and significant way. But, are we trusting Him with our valley experiences? We spend so much time praying that we don't end up in a valley, that we don't realize the knowledge that can be gained there. We tend to want to graduate with honors, without the knowledge we get from attending and taking part in class.

Valley experiences can be difficult, but they are necessary. The key to those experiences is to learn the lesson. Once we learn the lesson, we can move from there, equipped with the knowledge we gained.

Valleys most often have rivers and streams flowing through them. There is substance there in the valley; there is life there. We are provided for in the valley. God does not drop us there, and then leave us; He lives right there with us.

Let's embrace the experience, learn from it, and then grow from there. Then, we get to rejoice from the mountaintop.

Reflection

What if I told you that the Universe is conspiring to give you everything you need?

We spend so much time worrying about the trivial things, not realizing that everything we need is within our grasp. Our thoughts, words and actions are the key to it all.

The Universe is within us.

By making the powerful decision to take this journey to wellness and wholeness, you are making yourself part of that conspiracy. Only greatness can come of it.

Before you get started, take a moment to reflect on what you hope to gain from this journey. Where is your brokenness? Identify your scars, the obvious ones and the ones only visible to you. Over the course of our journey, we will learn to make peace with our brokenness, our wounds, our scars.

...and so, our journey begins.

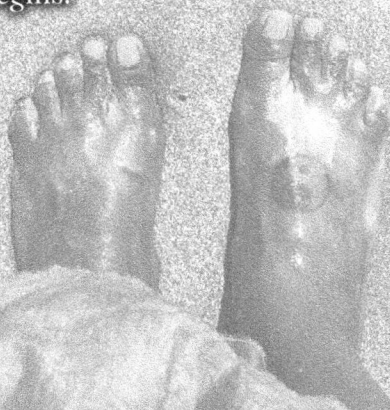

Chapter 8

———— ✳ ————

Healing the Sacred Womb

To say that healing the womb is essential would be an understatement. Womb healing restores our energy, removes emotional and spiritual blockages, releases us from spiritual strongholds and brings balance between our physical body and our spiritual body.

Womb healing is necessary for every woman, no matter her circumstances. We each spent months inside of our own mother's womb; our mother spent months in her mother's womb – and this traces back to the beginning of our families' lineages. Every bit of ancestral hurt ever felt by any woman in our lineage created an imprint on the inhabitants of her womb. That imprint was passed on to every descendant, including us. For women whose ancestors were in bondage, this can create havoc on our spirit. We carry the emotional and energetic wounds of every woman that came before us. We MUST heal the sacred womb!

I have had womb healing clients come to me for a womb blessing. A womb blessing is done using energy healing -similar to what you would see with Reiki healing. This is a transformative experience which restores the sacred feminine and allows us to return to our authentic wholeness. In a place of authentic wholeness, we find like Dee, those attached to us are blessed as well.

"After my womb blessing, my relationship with my husband improved dramatically. I was also able to reconnect with my mother and forgive her for years of emotional and physical abuse. My entire life was transformed after my womb blessing session. Every woman must do this for themselves and their families."

The womb has a memory. Unless we allow ourselves to heal, we will continue to pass down a legacy of brokenness. We are not healing for ourselves alone, we are healing for them too.

LET'S GET THE
WHEELS MOVING

Chapter 9

———— ✳ ————

Clearing the Path

There are several paths to this journey, so many components involved with healing. Chakras are a suitable place to start. Chakras are the seven spiritual, energetic centers within our bodies. Chakra is a Sanskrit word that simply means "wheel." Imagine these seven important wheels keeping everything moving and flowing. When the wheels need maintenance, movement is prohibited and a feeling of stuckness(my word) is created; in the same way you would be stuck if the wheels on your vehicle did not work. Each chakra has its own purpose and function, and although they are independent in nature, they are dependent in function. To feel whole, complete, healthy and well, all seven wheels must be operational and functioning at their full capacity.

The first chakra is at the base of the spine. The chakras travel upwards from there, through the abdominal area, the heart, the throat, all the way to the crown of our head. In order, our chakras are the Root (also known as the Base), Sacral, Solar Plexus, Heart, Throat, Third Eye and Crown. Each is symbolized by its own color and symbol, and has its own meaning, purpose, nature of healing and methods of remaining healthy. The chakra wheels being fully functional, allow for movement of chi throughout our bodies. Good chi is essential to our physical and emotional well-being.

WHAT THE HECK IS CHI?

Chi is a Greek word, but to understand chi, we should look to Chinese medicine. Chi is our life force; our energy flow. Imagine that chi is the highway that our soul, spirit and body use to connect, communicate and interact with each other. Chinese medicine teaches that to achieve and support physical and emotional health, chi must be allowed to freely flow throughout the human body. To have good chi, we must create an environment around us and within ourselves where this can occur. Good chi will bring balance within the body, and this is essential to our physical and emotional well-being.

There are several reasons why chi would not be able to flow freely within us. Fibroid tumors presented obstacles for me, but even after they were gone, I needed to heal that toxic energy within me. My body had been a toxic dump for so long; I needed more than surgery to clear that up. Heartbreak, physical and mental illness, the trauma associated with rape, sexual abuse and misuse; these are just a few examples of what can block the flow of good chi.

The great news is this - even if you have been feeling stagnant due to chi not flowing freely within you - there are indeed methods for removing those blockages. There are many methods practitioners use to help their patients restore good chi. What I designed for my healing, and now I share with you are the methods I used to restore myself after years of painful moon cycles, womb trauma, a hysterectomy and the loss of my sense of self.

Chapter 10

———※———

Nature as Our Medicine

It is my belief that nature has provided us with many necessary components for healing. As we continue our journey from here, we will focus heavily on the use of crystals for healing the womb. But what exactly are crystals, and how do they help us heal? Crystals are beautiful, geometrical stones that form naturally in the earth. Crystals work by harnessing the energy from the earth, the sun and the moon. When we connect with a crystal for the purposes of healing, the energy from the stone positively interacts with the energetic fields within our bodies and bring us into alignment with nature, and our own natural state of being.

Crystals work best when we physically connect with them by holding them - or wearing them as jewelry. We can also connect with crystals indirectly by having them placed in various places throughout our homes.

Another key component to our healing is the use of essential oils. Essential oils are compounds extracted from the very essence of plants. Essential oils are effective when used as aromatherapy, or when placed on our skin. Essential oils can cause irritation when placed directly on the skin, so it is necessary to combine them with a heavier oil (carrier oil) such as olive oil, sunflower oil, jojoba oil, coconut oil, or another preferred oil of that type. It is important to note that it is safe to use 12 drops of essential oils for every fluid ounce of the carrier oil.

Reflection

Physical and chronic illness can contribute to our chi becoming stagnant, however our external environment can also be a factor. Trying to keep a relationship that has become toxic is like continually putting gasoline into a car with a fuel leak. It can be wasteful and explosive.

We will spend a lot of time on this journey focusing on our internal healing, but we cannot afford to allow our external environment to go unnoticed. Before we go any further, take inventory of the people around you. Have they allowed you to create an environment that promotes your healing, or are they part of what you need to be healed from?

Walking away from a relationship, even one that has become toxic can be difficult. I can assure you from my own experience that it is not only possible, but it is essential to your journey.

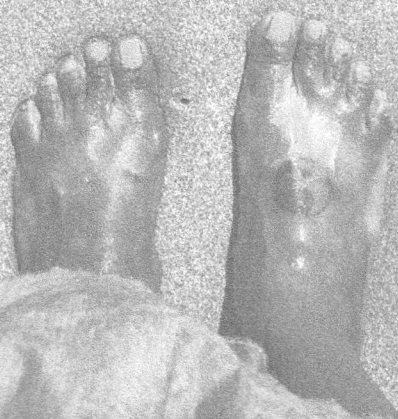

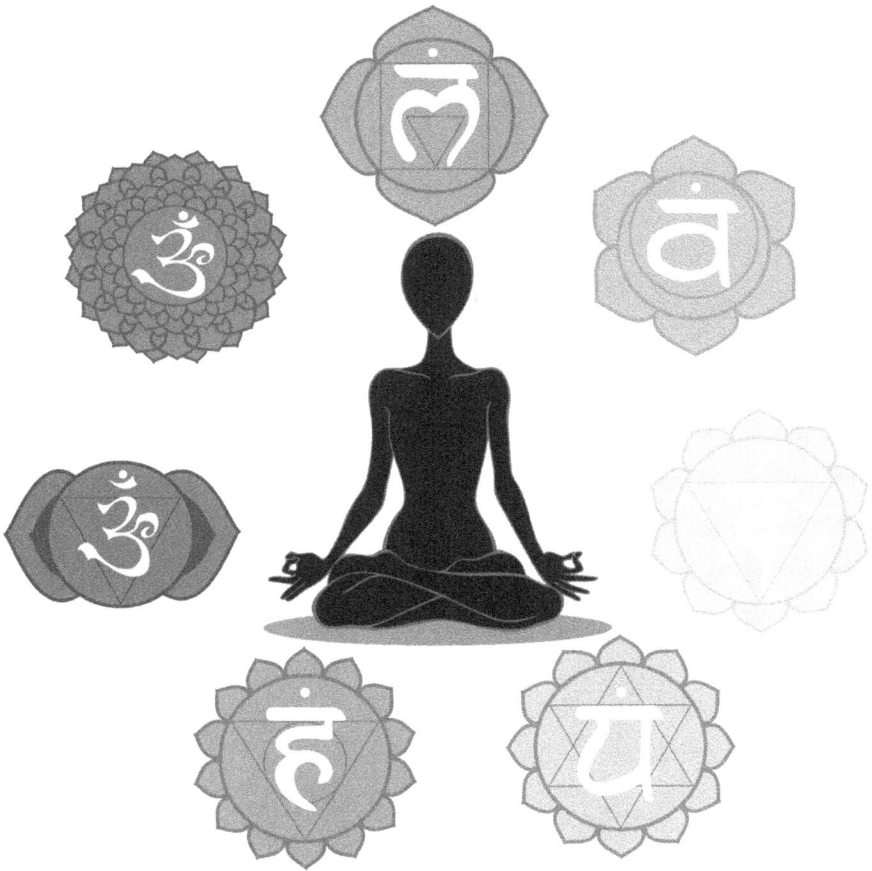

Chapter 11

---※---

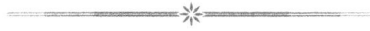

In Your Healing Box

As we begin, I will mention various elements used in the healing process. For your convenience, here are a few tools to have on hand for this leg of the journey...

Crystals: (at least one of the following; but as many as you choose):
Tiger's eye
Ruby
Smoky quartz
Rose quartz
Garnet

It is important that you choose a stone that you are attracted to - so choose wisely. There are many brick and mortar stores available to find an array of stones, but they can also be purchased online.

Incense or Essential oils:
Patchouli
Myrrh (yes, like the one from the Bible)
Lavender

Water: this is essential for every chakra.

Foods:

A green diet (kale, spinach, broccoli) is essential to a healthy womb. Root Vegetables are also vital and intentional as we focus on the Root Chakra. These include beets, carrots, sweet potatoes, turnips, are all among my favorites.

Although some of the tools will change from chakra to chakra, the methods of use may be similar

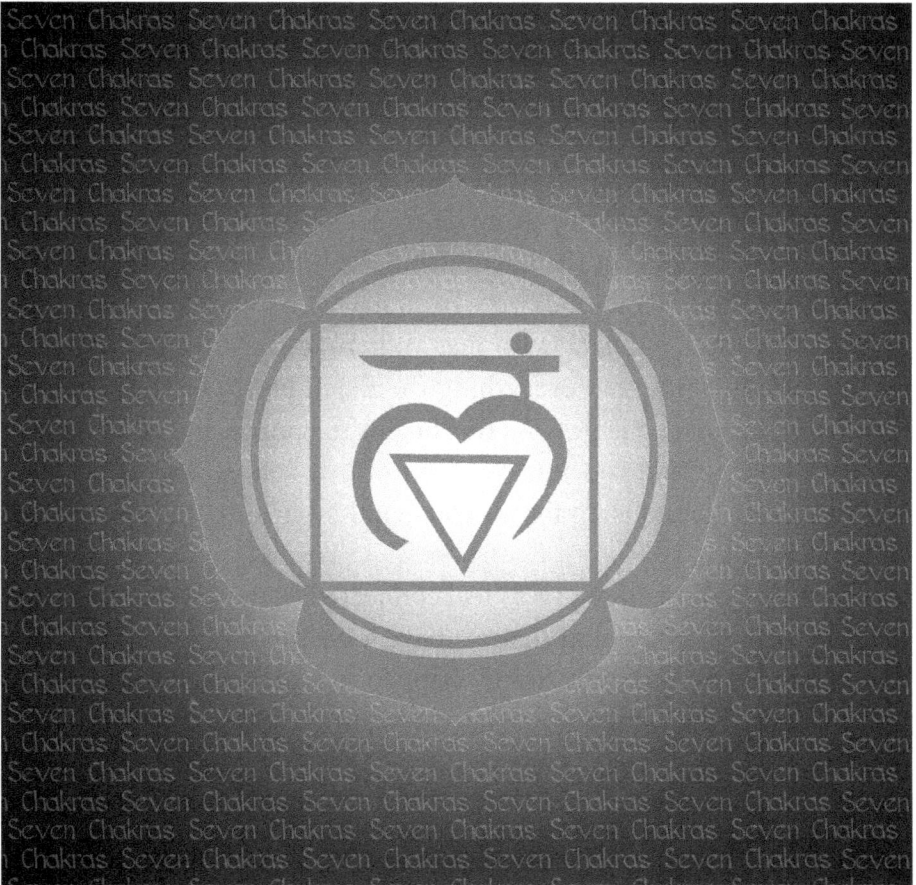

Chapter 12

---※---

Getting to the Root of the Matter

"There is a shade of red for every woman." Audrey Hepburn, Actress

To begin the process of healing, we must start at the beginning. The Sanskrit word for the first chakra is Muladhara, which means "root" or "support." The Root Chakra is associated with the color red and symbolized by a lotus flower with four petals. For healing the womb, and restoring our chi, we need to start at the Root Chakra. Have you ever heard the term "getting grounded?" This is where that takes place. Everything we need is in the Earth; from the minerals our bodies need, to the nutritional plants that grow from it.

Stand up for a moment with just your bare feet on the ground. I want you to imagine that everything the Earth has to offer is entering your body through your feet. As this begins to happen and all of Earth's energy begins to find you, it travels up towards your torso. At the base of your torso; the housing for all your vital organs, there is your Root Chakra.

The Root Chakra allows us to feel connected to the Earth; connected to ourselves. It is essential that we have a healthy Root Chakra. This is not something that will simply happen, we must make allowances for it. There are several ways to have a healthy and freely moving Root Chakra.

Chapter 13

***

Let's Get Grounded!

Getting grounded is essential to our journey of wellness and wholeness. Being grounded means to be fully present in your body, while feeling connected with the Earth and its elements.

Imagine trying to build a house without a solid foundation. Anything you build on it will surely collapse. This is the same with our Root Chakra; we cannot begin to balance the remaining chakras until we have strengthened our base.

Many years ago, I started this whole phase of walking outside barefoot. I really did not worry about how dirty the ground was. I did not have an intellectual reason for choosing to walk around outdoors barefoot, but it certainly felt right for me. Even without knowing why I was doing it, I was getting grounded. Now when I walk barefoot outdoors, I do so with purpose and intent. This is where I want you to start.

Go outside, find a place where it is just you and the ground; no concrete or asphalt. This area can be a mound of dirt, sand or grass. Take your shoes off and stand there. Awe! I want you to focus on what that feels like. Focus on nothing else except the way you feel standing there, connected to the Earth. Be present in that moment.

As you stand there, barefoot on the ground, I want you to say these words. "I am connected, I am present." Say that as many times as you need to until you feel connected and present. This is something I encourage you to do as often as you need it.

YOU ARE STARTING THE PROCESS OF GETTING GROUNDED AND ROOTED. IT JUST GETS BETTER FROM HERE.

Meditation is essential to getting grounded. Meditating is an avenue you can use to incorporate other aspects of healing, such as crystals, sacred smoke and affirmations. There are several positions used for the purpose of meditating, but the most common, and certainly the most effective method for grounding is the Sukhasana pose; also known as the easy pose. There are several poses effective for grounding while meditating, but this one is an easy go-to for starting.

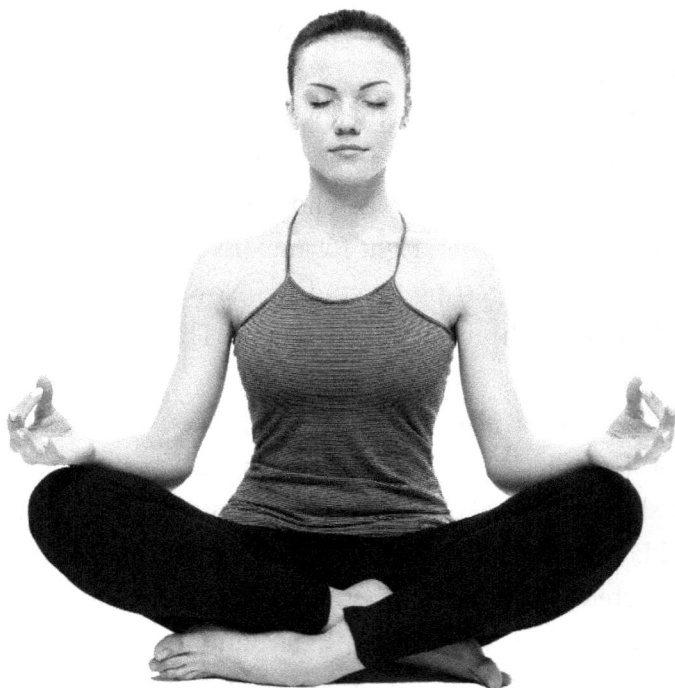

This pose allows you to sit on the Earth with your Root Chakra to the ground. This method of grounding goes straight to source. Meditating in this way is extremely beneficial and effective for several reasons. In addition to the grounding benefits this offers, the act of meditation itself, has a whole slew of benefits. Meditation helps reduce stress, helps control anxiety, increases self-awareness, and allows you to focus on the present. This is essential to your journey.

Meditating in this method will allow you to use your crystals. While sitting in Sukhasana, your hands should be open, facing upwards, as if you are expecting to be handed a gift. This is a brilliant way of holding your crystals. This method of mediation will be used at every chakra level, and the crystal you hold in your hand should align with the chakra you are focusing on. At this stage, we are focused on the Root Chakra, and the stones should be associated with it. I love using the Rose quartz for root chakra meditating, but you can use any stone associated with this area. Find a crystal that you connect with, and let that stone be the one you use for your Root Chakra meditation.

Mediation is also an ideal time to burn your incense. (As we move upwards towards the Crown Chakra, you will be introduced to more conduits of sacred smoke.) In many cultures, smoke is used to connect with and communicate with the divine spirit. Incense is also used all throughout the Bible. When Aaron needed to communicate with God, he took burning coal and incense with him (Leviticus 16:12). Smoke is considered sacred, and it is believed that the smoke elevates your prayers, affirmations and meditative thoughts into the Universe, and right to the heart of God. Grounding meditation offers yet another opportunity for saying your affirmations, beginning with "I am connected, I am present."

"Let food be thy medicine and medicine be thy food." Hippocrates, The Father of Medicine.

How many times have you heard the saying, "you are what you eat?" This is true. What we eat becomes a part of us. The nutrients we get from our healthy foods, or the toxins we get from our unhealthy foods. It is essential that we watch what we place inside of our bodies as it certainly does enter the bloodstream; and our blood travels everywhere throughout our bodies, through every vital organ. This is something I came to appreciate after I got sick.

Anemia is a common disorder for a woman with fibroids in her uterus. It can also be significant in women who have heavy moon cycles. Anemia can cause a low hemoglobin level, and a low hemoglobin level is dangerous. During the period after I was hospitalized in December of 2016, and underwent my hysterectomy in January of 2017, I was tasked with taking care of myself, as the fibroids were still living inside of me. It was during this time that I was introduced to Dr. Peter J. D'Adamo's book, "Eat Right for Your Type." This book teaches the importance of learning your blood type and eating according to it. Dr. D'Adamo teaches that each blood type is unique, and so how we feed our blood needs to be unique to our type. Through this book I learned that some foods act as medicine to us, some foods acts as poison, and some foods simply act as food.

For someone with a blood disorder, eating foods that are medicinal are beneficial to our health. Eating foods that are not can cause illnesses to occur. For the month leading up to my surgery, I ate only the foods that were considered beneficial, and I can assure you it works. When I left the hospital on the evening of December 27, 2016 after having several blood transfusions, my hemoglobin level had been elevated to 7.5. On the morning of January 27, 2017 (just one-month later), after having my hemoglobin level checked in pre-op, it was at 12.5. The only thing I had done differently within that one -month, was eat the foods that were beneficial to my blood type. This included a greener diet.

There are many foods that I found essential for grounding. During this phase of our chakra healing, we should begin to eat foods that are directly connected to the Earth. This would include a plant-based diet, as well as root vegetables. I did not need rocket science knowledge to understand this; eating foods that came from the Earth would allow me to connect with the Earth.

Everyone should speak with their own physician about a nutritional diet, however, my meals consisted of a lot of raw and cooked greens, roasted sweet potato fries seasoned with Himalayan salt and cayenne pepper, and other nutritious foods. I also fell madly in love with juicing; combining beets, carrots, apple and a little ginger. It is essential to eat foods that are rich in Earth's minerals. This is beneficial for both our emotional and physical health.

Affirmations:
"I am grounded."
"I am connected to the earth beneath me."
"I am safe."

Reflection

    Today, practice the art of disconnecting in order that you might reconnect. Take time for yourself. Go for a walk-in nature. If you live in a coastal area, go for a walk along the beach; let your feet connect with the ocean. If you live near the mountains, go for a short hike. If you live near a park, grab a blanket, a book, and your favorite treats, and have a solo picnic. Take your shoes off, let your feet connect with the ground beneath you.

    This is a perfect time for grounding, relaxation and rejuvenation.

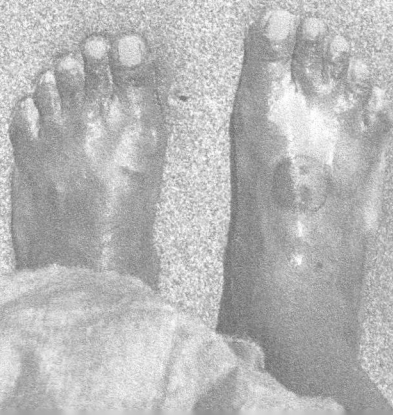

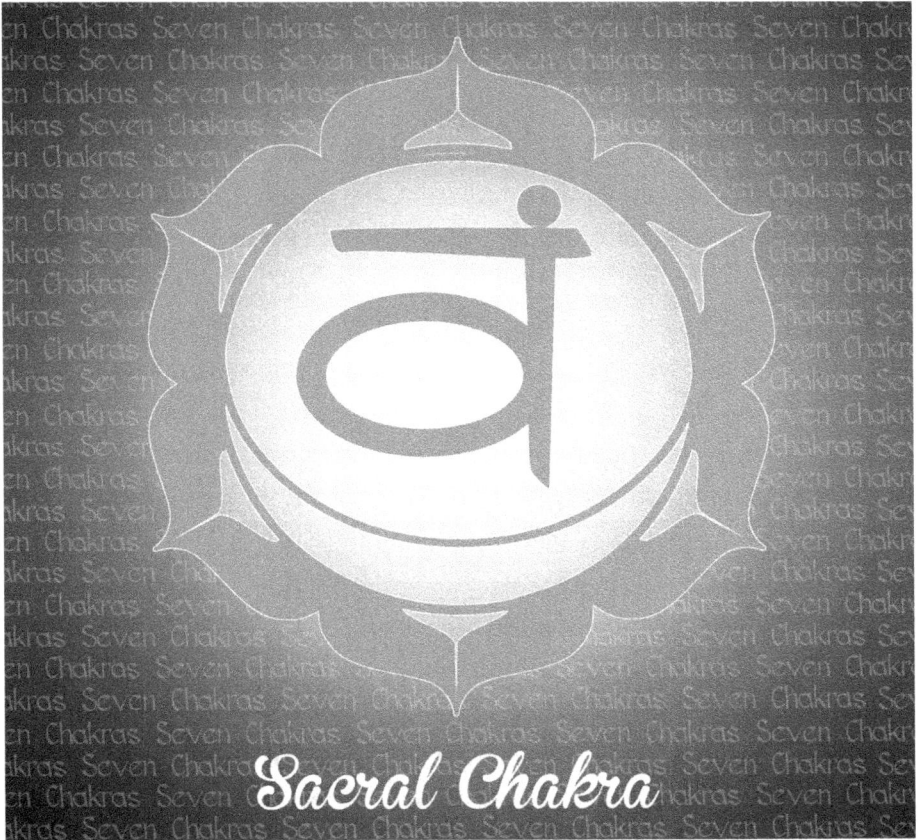

Sacral Chakra

Chapter 14

---❈---

The Sweet Spot

"Orange is the happiest color." Frank Sinatra, Singer

As we journey through healing our chakras, the next stop is the sweet spot. The Sanskrit word for the second chakra is Svadhisthana, which means "sweetness." The Sacral Chakra is the place of pleasure for us. This is where we find our sexuality and our carnal pleasure. The Sacral Chakra is represented by a six petalled lotus flower and associated with the color orange. Water is the element associated with this chakra.

In the same way we had certain tools we needed when working on our Root Chakra, we will need tools for this leg of our journey.

The Crystals we need for balancing our Sacral Chakra include: Golden Topaz and Citrine. These are two of my favorite stones. You can also use Carnelian. Again, it is essential that you choose a stone that you are attracted to, because you will certainly spend a lot of time with it. The incense and essential oils needed are Jasmine, Sandalwood and Rose. Water is essential for every chakra, but especially this one, as this chakra requires a lot of liquids. Color plays such a huge part in balancing our chakras, so for the purpose of the Sacral Chakra, I think orange juice would be essential. In addition to orange juice, because greens are so important for womb health, the Sacral Chakra is a wonderful time to introduce green smoothies. YUM!

Green smoothies are so delicious, especially when done right. There are various recipes for the perfect green smoothie, but my favorite includes kale, a little spinach, water, chia or flax seeds, pineapple (extremely beneficial) blueberries and sweetened with honey. Another liquid-based meal would be a yogurt smoothie using a nut milk (almond is my favorite) and fruit. Drink lots of water!

It is essential to balance the Sacral Chakra. When this chakra is unbalanced, we feel disconnected from our sexuality, and can lose all desire in that area of our lives. If you are going through a season of purposeful celibacy, this may not be a huge deal to you; but for everyone else this can be huge. In addition to a loss of sexual desire, an unbalanced Sacral Chakra can cause issues with our bladder and lower back. An unbalance here could also bring emotional imbalance.

Meditation is essential with every chakra, and our methods are the same. When meditating for the purpose of the Sacral Chakra, we will use the proper crystals and use the appropriate scents. There are several affirmations that can be used for this chakra, and you should feel free to customize your own. For those who need a little shove, I offer you this one. "I am happy and fulfilled. I am enough." Say this as many times as you need to until it resonates within your beautiful spirit. "I am happy and fulfilled. I am enough."

The Sacral Chakra is also the chakra that controls our creativity and our passion. When I speak here of passion, I am not referring to it in a sexual sense, but in the sense of being passionate about something, the way a chef is passionate about food. If you are an artist of any kind, the Sacral Chakra is the birthplace of your creativity. As a writer, having a balanced Sacral Chakra is essential to my purpose.

"Healing the Womb…" seems like such a crazy title for a book written by a woman who has no physical womb. The womb, however, is as much a spiritual space as it is a physical. Men also have spiritual wombs, even though they do not have a physical one. For me, healing the womb was about getting back to what made me, me.

ALLOW ME TO GET REALLY PERSONAL.

In the weeks following my hysterectomy, I dealt with serious fears. In addition to feeling disconnected from my sexuality, I felt disconnected from my creativity. I struggled to recognize myself, and I started to withdraw from all the things I had once been connected with. I felt as if I had lost my voice (we will discuss this a little more when we get to the fifth chakra). My publisher reached out to me, hopeful that I would write a book (this book) about my experience. How could I write a book? I had no creative voice, and I was still trying to figure out how to heal myself. I could not begin to help others while I was still struggling to understand it all.

In my research, I kept coming across something I don't recall ever hearing about previously. The Yoni egg!

CAN WE TALK ABOUT COOKIES?

Yoni, like chakra is a Sanskrit word. Yoni translates to womb. Yoni is the Hindu word for our vagina; our sacred space; the cookie; the good stuff; the sweet spot (ok, I'll stop).

The Yoni egg is a smooth crystal, shaped like an egg for the purpose of insertion into our vaginas. Discovering this little nugget was so essential to my healing. The Yoni egg is available in several crystal varieties, but I found Jade and Rose Quartz are the most popular. After doing some research, I decided to go with the Jade stone because of the benefits Jade offers.

The most common color of Jade is green. Jade has many benefits, it is effective for emotional healing as it helps alleviate anxiety and brings harmony. Rose Quartz has amazing qualities, and it is a stone I use a lot, but when searching for a Yoni egg, I felt Jade was better suited for my purposes. The Yoni egg will be the stone that you are most intimate with (for obvious reasons), therefore it is so important that you choose the right one.

The Yoni egg is essential for healing the womb. Using a Yoni egg has several benefits, as it awakens our sensuality as well as our sexuality. It allows us to feel connected with ourselves; essential if like me, you felt/ feel disconnected. The Yoni egg increases our sex drive and it facilitates an enjoyable sexual experience. The Yoni egg can improve our overall sense of well-being. For women who are experiencing womb trauma due to natural childbirth, you may find using the Yoni egg beneficial for strengthening the pelvic muscle.

The Yoni egg comes in three varied sizes - small, medium and large. When ordering them online, they usually come as a set, allowing you to make the decision through trial and error. For most women, it will either be the medium egg, for women who have had more than one vaginal birth, the larger egg may be the perfect fit. It is necessary to physically clean the egg when you receive it. The Yoni egg should be gently hand washed using warm water and a mild, unscented hypoallergenic soap. After you have washed your egg, it is essential to clear the energy of the egg. This is done through a sage smudge.

Light your sage, wait for the fire to burn out (you can blow it out as well) and allow the smoke to permeate the Yoni egg. This is essential to clearing the energy of everyone who handled the egg before you bought it.

Be sure to place your burning or smoking sage inside of a flame-retardant dish. This method of clearing the energy of a gemstone can be used with all your crystals.

The Yoni egg will come with two small holes drilled into it. These holes are for adding string. The string is helpful when removing the egg from the vagina. Some eggs will come pre-strung, but if not, you can use floss or a thick thread.

The Yoni egg is inserted in the same way in which you would a tampon. To remove it, simply relax your pelvic muscle and pull out. Clean your egg after you remove it.

The first few times you use the Yoni egg, you will certainly be aware of its presence. Over time, some women will get use to the way it feels and may not think about it until it is time to remove it at the end of the day. Others may be aware of its presence every moment of the day. Even for the most timid amongst us, it may feel natural over time and you may even begin to feel like your Yoni egg is a part of you.

LET'S VENTURE MORE INTO THE YONIVERSE

Losing your sex drive after a hysterectomy can be quite normal. The removal of your ovaries can result in a decrease in the libido and this loss of sex drive can be furthered by hysterectomy - promoted instant menopause. After my procedure, I felt completely disconnected from my sexuality. I had little to no interest in sex or intimacy. A large part of it had to do with my emotional imbalance, additionally, I felt less of a woman. I felt like the pathway between me and my vagina had been blocked and I no longer viewed myself as a sexual being.

When I began to use the yoni egg, I felt the pathway clearing. Having the egg inserted in my yoni and being aware of its presence caused me to focus more on that area of my body. It did not take long before I felt reconnected to my sexuality.

Prior to using the yoni egg, I felt completely void of sexual thoughts. After using it, my sex drive went through the roof. Instead of a loss of libido, I felt a complete surge of sexuality, and when I found the right sexual partner, I was unstoppable! Aside from the healing properties of the stone itself, I believe that the yoni egg is powerful in that it forces us to focus more on our vagina and the pleasures that can exist there. I find that even when I do not have the yoni egg inserted, just the visual of it allows me to focus on my happy place.

IT'S ALL ELEMENTARY MY DEAR.

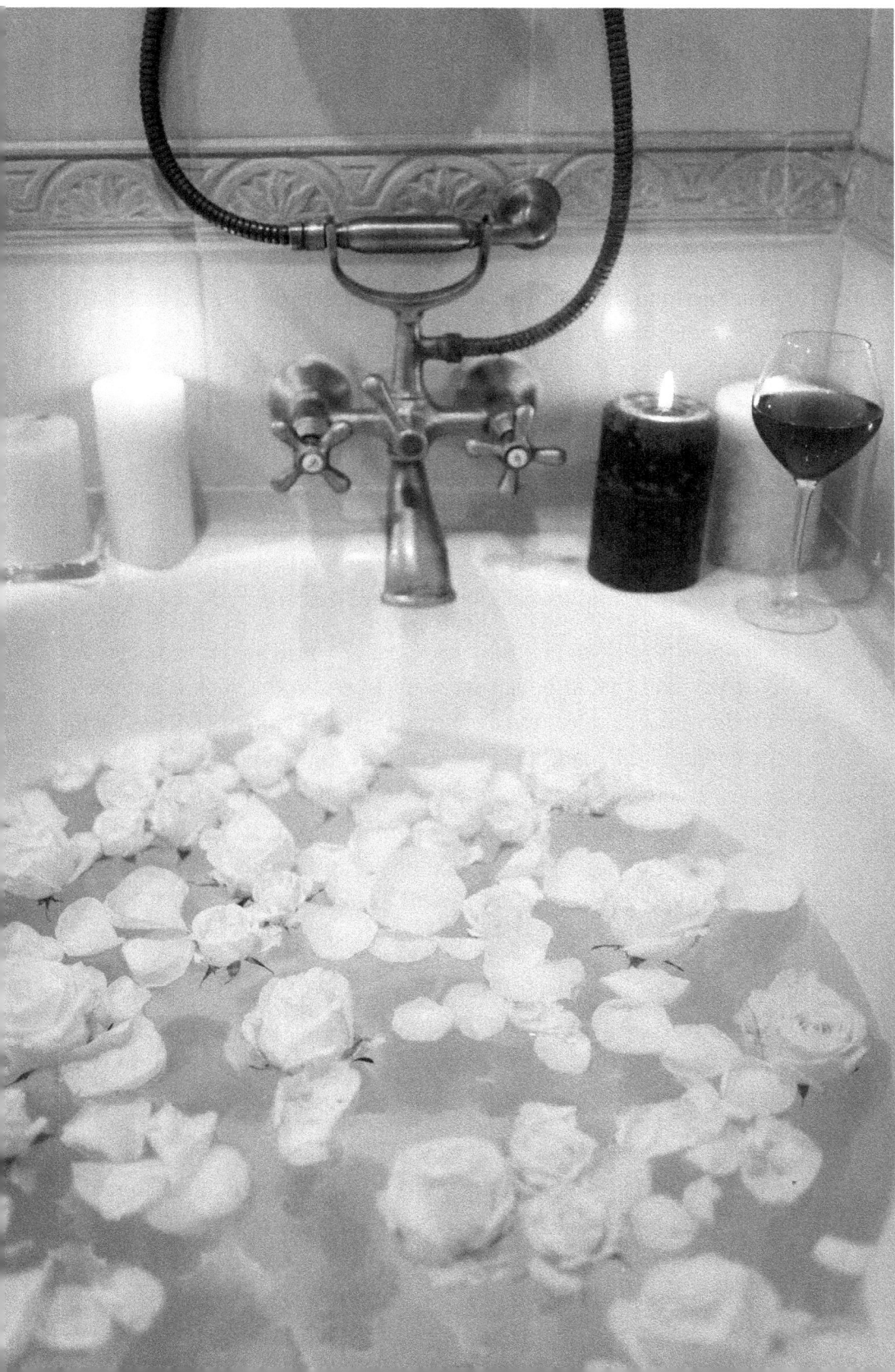

Since the element for the Sacral Chakra is water, this is a wonderful time to treat yourself to what I call "The Goddess Bath." This method of bathing is one of the first, purposeful things I did when I began my journey of wellness and wholeness, and I continue to do this.

To understand the spiritual significance of bathing, we can look back to early Jewish tradition. Mikveh is a Jewish ritual bath. Traditionally, a woman would immerse in a mikveh in preparation for marriage and after her monthly cycle. This ritual is about cleanliness and restoration. The Goddess bath comes from this tradition, but with some other additives.

The Goddess bath is so essential to restoring the sacred feminine. You can customize it to safely fit your needs, but I created a recipe that works best for me and I would love to share that with you.

Starting with a clean bathtub, run water as warm as you can tolerate; keeping in mind that although we want to warm the cookie, we don't want to bake the cookie. Add a generous amount (about 10 drops each) of the essential oils: lavender, frankincense and geranium. Toss in a generous amount of organic lavender and rose buds (easily bought online) and light some candles. Some might say that the candles are optional, but I think they are mandatory. I am usually a proponent of scented candles, but trust me girlfriend, your Goddess bath, filled with those essential oils and flower buds, has all the fragrance you'll need.

Use this time of mikveh to focus only on your healing. Do your affirmations, read a self-help book (not this one, you don't want this one getting wet), drink water (it gets hot in there), listen to music. Sit back, relax and enjoy.

The Sacral Chakra is all about flow. When focusing on healing this chakra, this is what you must do: remain fluid - remain open-minded to your healing and listen to what your body tells you. The Sacral Chakra is the seat of our intuition, and you must learn to listen to it.

FISH FOOD FOR THOUGHT

If you feel stuck or stagnant and don't feel your creative or sexual juices flowing (pun intended), take the advice of that whacky blue fish, Dory, (Finding Dory and Finding Nemo, Disney/Pixar movies) jump in a large body of water and "just keep swimming."

Affirmations:
"I am a creative spirit. My life is my art."
"I am sexually vibrant."
"I am whole."

Reflection

On this journey, it is important to be Goddess enough to rise above the nonsense that exists in our world, but human enough to remain grounded.

Disconnect – purposefully - as often as you need to. Escape into the Goddess Bath as often as you see fit. There is no appointed time. There are moments when you will feel stagnant, despite your best efforts. That is okay. You are building the tools you need to bounce back as often as you need to.

We will no longer be defined by our brokenness, but by our ability to heal and make it look effortless.

You are a Goddess! You got this!

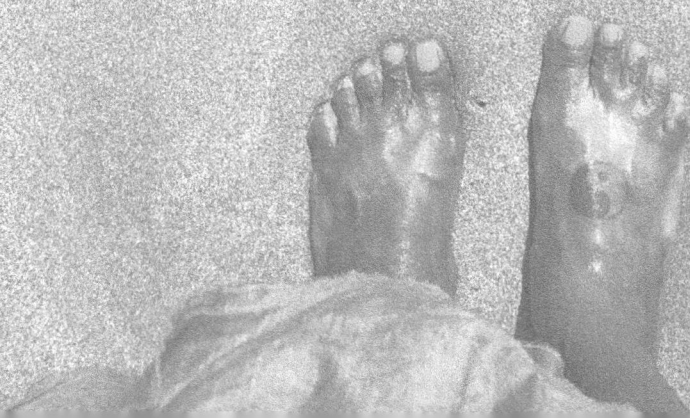

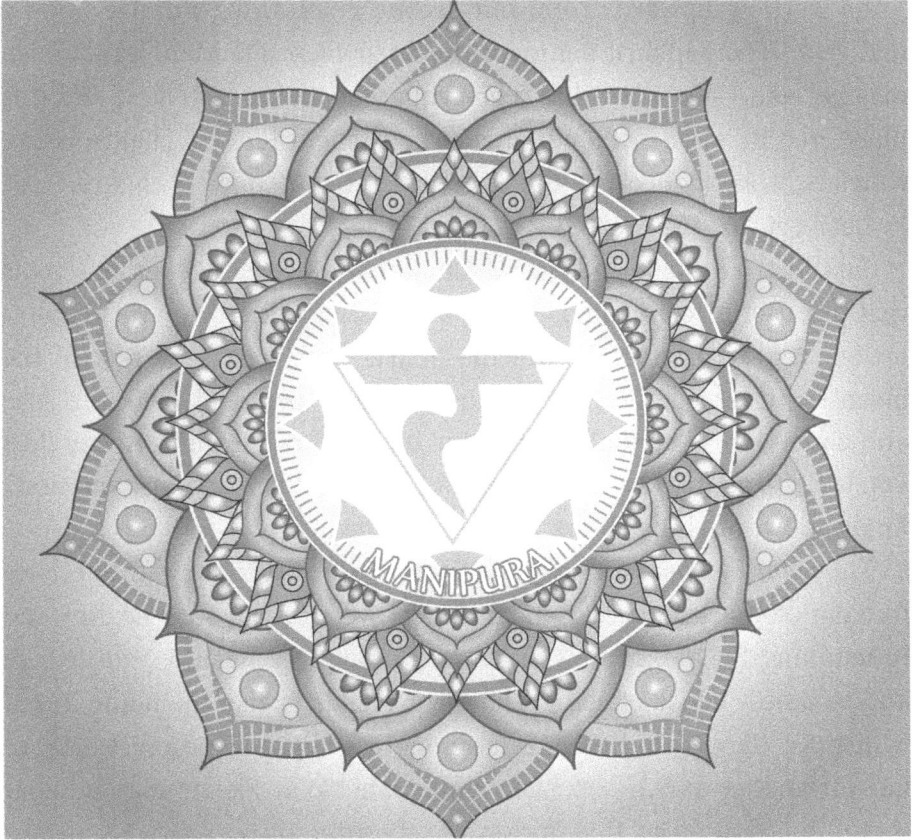

Chapter 15

---※---

Hey There Sunshine!

"I really just want to be warm yellow light that pours over everyone I love." Conor Oberst, Singer-Songwriter

As we flow upwards from our second chakra, we stumble upon a real gem. The Sanskrit name for the Solar Plexus is Manipura, which means "gem." The color that represents this chakra is yellow, and it is illustrated by a ten-petalled lotus. The element for this chakra is fire which is probably because this is considered our "power" chakra.

Let's get this fire started.

Just like our Root and Sacral Chakras, the Solar Plexus has tools that are useful for balancing it. The crystals needed for this chakra include Yellow citrine, Aventurine quartz and Topaz. A few of the incense and essential oils are ylang ylang (a personal favorite), rose and cinnamon. The food needed for this chakra's health are starches. Potatoes being my favorite and one of the healthier options; and don't forget to hydrate! It gets hot in the Solar Plexus.

The Solar Plexus is found just below your rib cage; this is the area we find our stomach, pancreas and digestive system. Having a healthy and functioning Solar Plexus is essential to having a healthy self-esteem and a healthy sense of self. The Solar Plexus is also the home to our willpower. If you find that you are one who likes to procrastinate, or has difficulties staying on task, a stagnant Solar Plexus may be your issue. In addition to this, if you are the type of person who always feels victimized as if others are responsible for your bad luck; polish your gem!

GET EMPOWERED!

I LOVE sunflowers. They are like beautiful little suns in a vase. They really do have a way of brightening up a space, and I cannot understand how anyone could come into contact with sunflowers and walk away unhappy. In addition to being absolutely radiant, they can be quite beneficial.

Sunflower oil is rich in vitamins A, C and D and it has regenerative properties. You may already know that you can use sunflower oil for cooking, but what if I told you that it makes a great base for a "Goddess Oil."

IF YOU THOUGHT THE GODDESS BATH WAS AMAZING, WAIT TILL YOU GET A HOLD OF THIS GEM.

I came up with this Goddess Oil as a way of making the Goddess Bath portable.

Using a travel size bottle, start with sunflower oil as your base. Add ylang ylang, cinnamon and frankincense. You can add other essential oils as well, according to your taste. My favorites include geranium and lavender. You can use this oil after your bath or shower; placing it on your feet, elbows and abdominal area. Use it generously, you can always make another batch when needed.

Affirmation:
"I am worthy, I am powerful. I am more than enough."

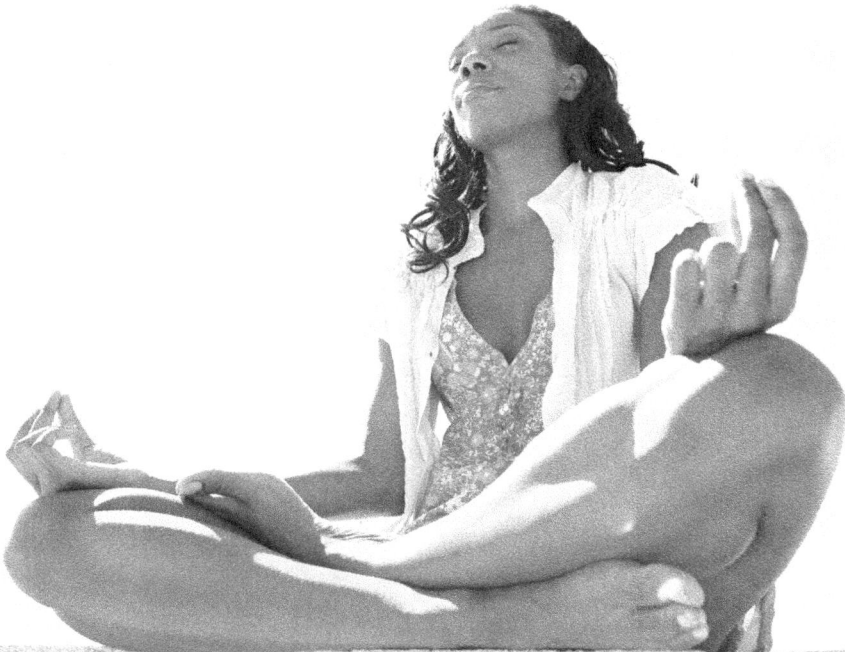

Reflection

I am what you might call an overthinker. This has caused me great anxiety. This is a daily journey for me.

One morning after one of my long nights, I was driving along the highway. I could not miss the Sun as she made her presence known up there in the sky. She got me to thinking; no matter what happened the night before, no matter how bad the storm, or dark the night, there she was, up there just shining! She is persistent.

That's just who she is.

She rises and shines every day without anyone's permission. Her light is so powerful; she supplies the moon's glow.

The same must be true of us. No matter what happened the night before, the morning brings new and fresh opportunities. We must be like the sun. We must shine through the dark clouds. We must rise despite last night's darkness. We need to be persistent, just like the sun. We need to supply enough light, that it lights the path for those who come after us.

We have more work to do; God is not finished with us yet. We have all made mistakes, a few bad choices and decisions. We have been purposefully rude, and a few times we were rude unintentionally. We have been naive about some choices, and other times, we have been methodical. Regardless of the situation, the new day provides us with a new opportunity for correction.

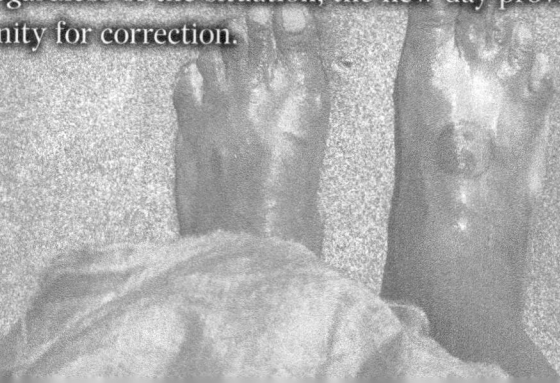

Basking in the rays of the Sun

Let's get to the heart of the matter, as women, we are creatures of the Moon – the Moon borrows light from the Sun. There is something so incredible about allowing your body to purposely engage sunlight. Take a few moments and stand outside in the warmth of the day. Allow the sun to warm your beautiful skin. Take deep breaths – absorbing it all.

Open the curtains or the window coverings in your home. Allow the sunshine to come in and fill your home with natural and healing light. Your home is your sanctuary, and as you allow this light to permeate your home, it can also permeate your spirit.

Here is to a brand-new day!
We are on fire!

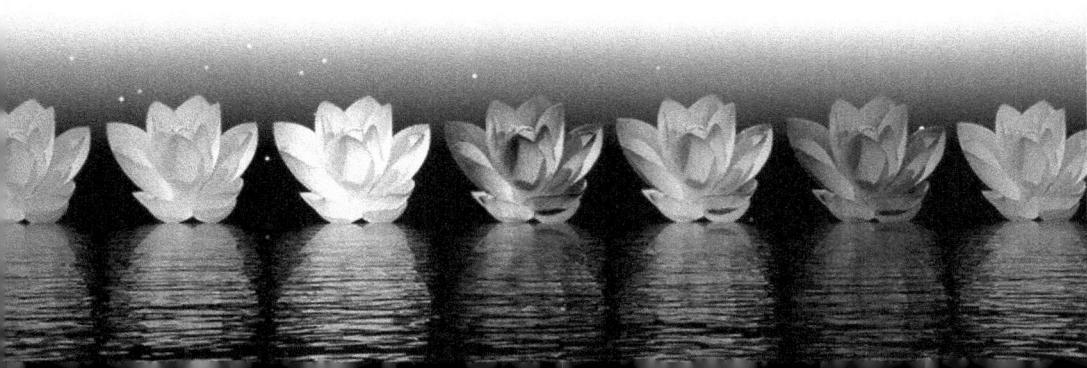

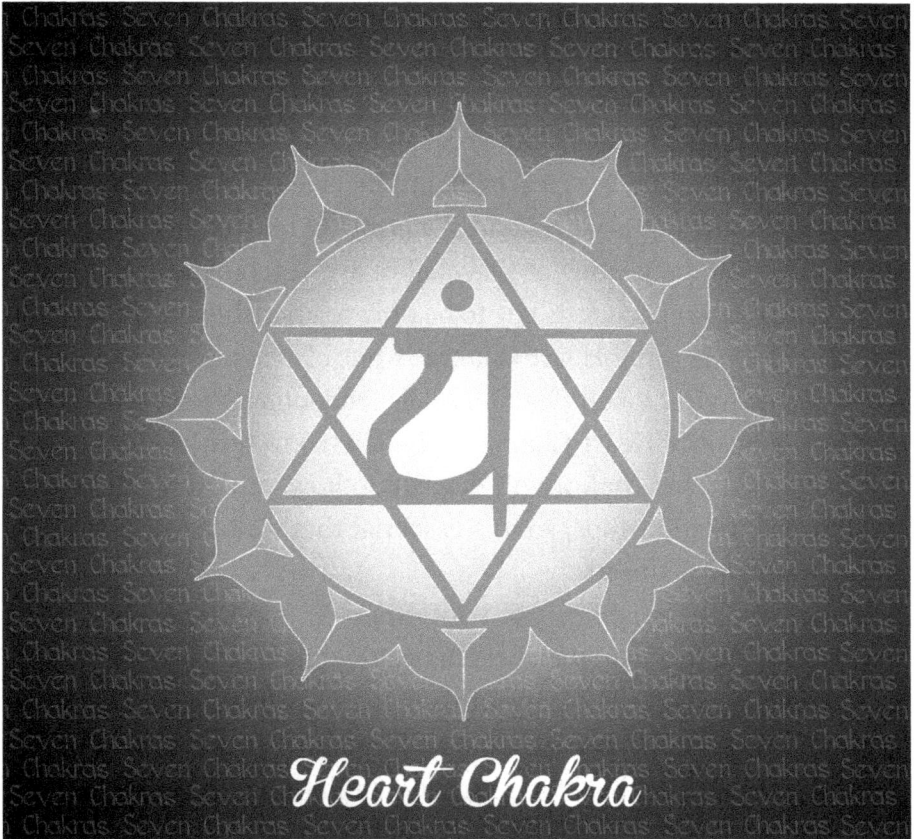

Heart Chakra

Chapter 16

Home is Where the Heart Is

"Green is the prime color of the world, and that from which its loveliness arises." Pedro Calderon de la Barca, Dramatist

The fourth chakra is Anahata, which in Sanskrit means "unstruck." This is our Heart Chakra. You ever had someone ask you, "where is the love?", well this is where it's at. The Heart Chakra is represented by a 12-petalled lotus, and the colors green and pink. The crystals used for balancing and healing the Heart Chakra include many of my favorites: jade, moonstone, Rose quartz and Watermelon tourmaline. The foods associated with the healing of this chakra are vegetables.

A healthy Heart Chakra is key to healthy relationships; with yourself, and others. When the Heart Chakra is out of balance or stagnant, it can cause us to feel lonely, fearful, co-dependent and betrayed. To the contrary, a healthy Heart Chakra will allow us to feel loved, accepted and balanced. This chakra will determine how you view friendships and intimate relationships, so it is essential that we take care of it and give it all the love it needs.

Having healthy relationships with others is important, but on this journey to wellness and wholeness, a healthy relationship with yourself is essential. As women, we spend so much time nurturing others, our self-care becomes secondary. This journey must be personal. This is a journey of personal healing, restoration and love. We cannot extend love to others while overlooking our own needs. A healthy relationship with self is essential to healthy relationships with others.

There is such a strong connection between the Heart Chakra and the womb. When our womb is used in the way that it was purposed: nurturing, creativity and birth, our Heart Chakra is strengthened, active and open. When our womb has become the toxic dumping ground for hurt, abuse and sickness, this weakens our Heart Chakra's ability to spin freely. Healing the womb then is essential to our quality of life and our quality of love – which flow from our heart.

SELF-CARE

Being selfish gets a bad rap, but there are times when it is necessary. This is one of those times, girl.

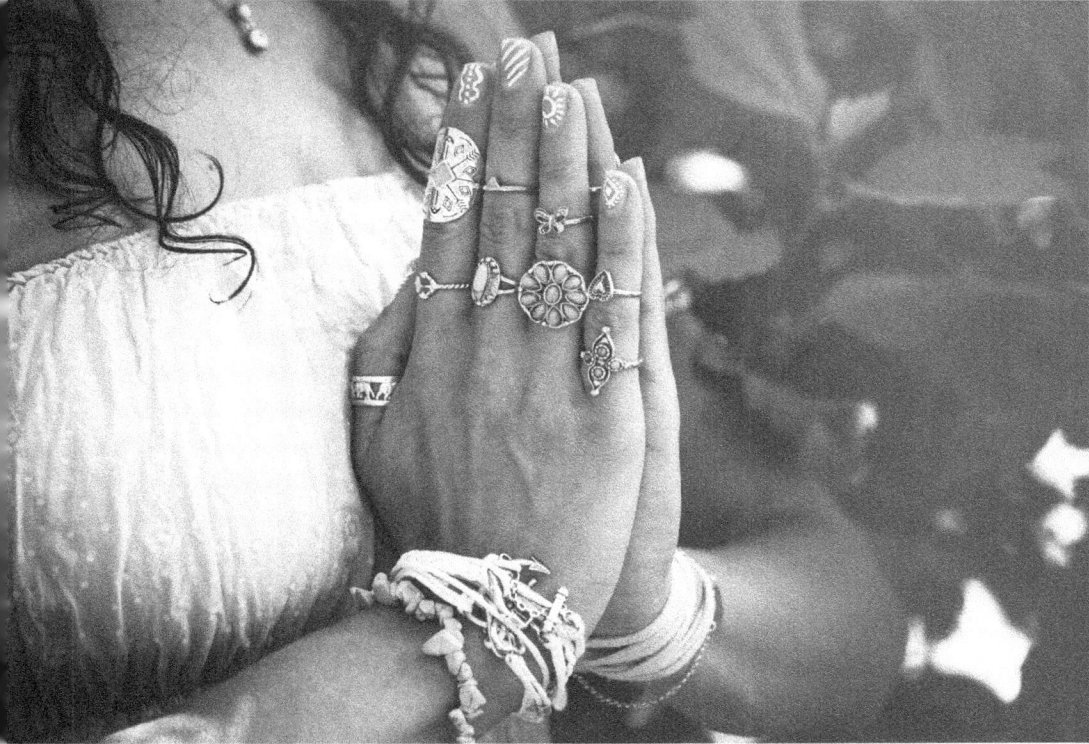

Affirmations:
"My heart is filled with love, for myself and for others."
"I love without condition, I am love."

Reflection

I spent most of life not knowing that my heart capacity could expand. Then I met a 2-year old little boy named John. I fell in love with him. I legally adopted him as my son.

Just when you think your heart has reached its capacity, God expands it, and makes room for more. Allow your heart the opportunity to expand. If there is someone you need to forgive, do that. Forgiveness expands the heart. Have you been considering getting a puppy? Scratch that idea, visit an animal shelter and adopt a dog. That dog is going to fall in love with you and you will fall in love too. Your heart will expand.

Every time we extend ourselves beyond what we thought was our full capacity, a miracle happens. Look for opportunities to do so. An open heart is a healthy and happy heart.

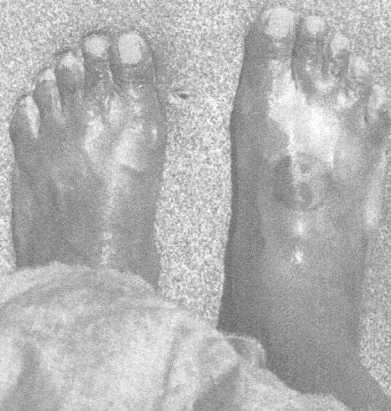

Each day brings its own possibilities. You wake up feeling refreshed, feeling like yourself again, and it is like the face in the mirror says, "welcome back!"

There are situations that occur in our lives that cause us to doubt our worth.

Today is the perfect day to remind yourself how utterly amazing you are.

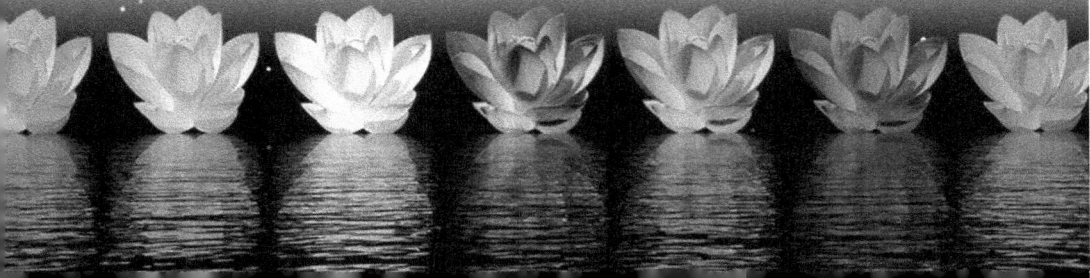

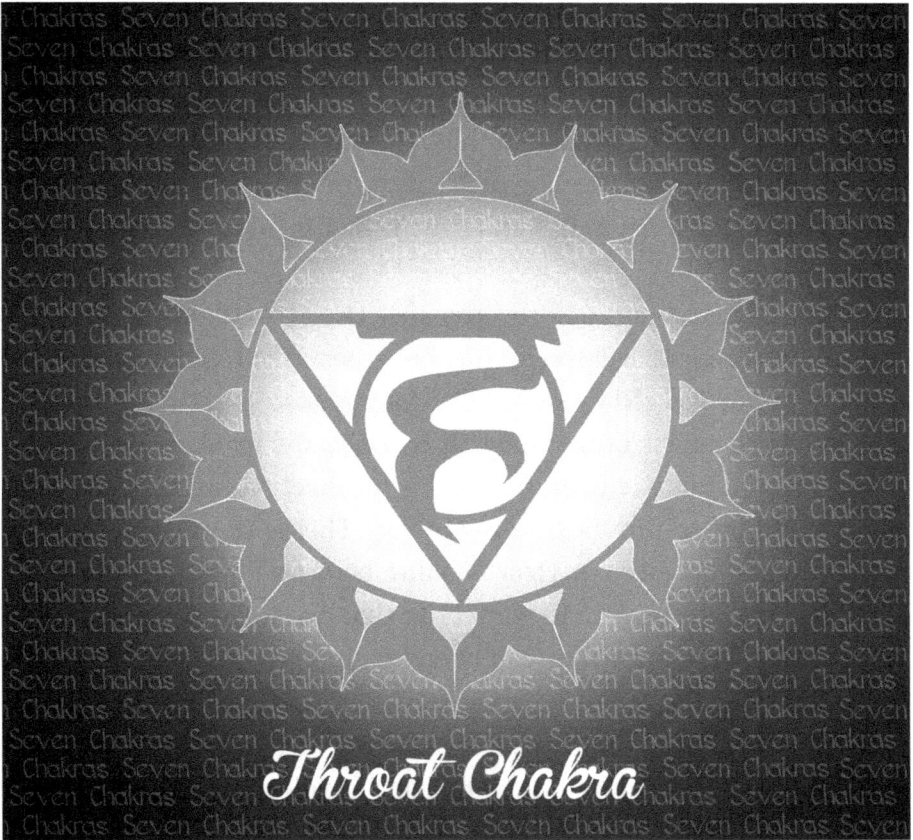

Throat Chakra

Chapter 17

---✳---

Can We Talk?

"Blue is the only color which maintains its own character in all its tones, it will always stay blue." Raoul Dufy, French painter

The Throat Chakra is our fifth chakra. The Sanskrit word for this chakra is Vishuddha which means "purity" and it is represented by the color blue. The lotus flower associate with the Throat Chakra has 16 petals; its element is Ether, a highly flammable and volatile liquid. We can imagine why the Throat Chakra, the place where are words are communicated from, has an element that is highly flammable and volatile.

In the biblical book of Proverbs 15:4 (NIV) we find these words, "the soothing tongue is a tree of life, but a perverse tongue crushes the spirit." James 3:6 (NIV) says, "The tongue also is a fire, a world of evil among the parts of the body. It corrupts the whole body, sets the whole course of one's life on fire, and is itself set on fire by hell." How can something so tiny be so disruptive? This is the reason why we must heal and balance our Heart Chakra before addressing our Throat Chakra. This ensures that the words that are formed come from a place of love; otherwise they can be quite disruptive. There is no room on this journey for chaos.

Fruit is beneficial for the Throat Chakra. I like to imagine that a piece of fruit can sweeten our words, and besides that, fruit has many important nutrients. The crystals associated with this chakra include Turquoise (my favorite), Sodalite. Agate, Sapphire and Aquamarine. Chamomile, with its soothing qualities and Myrrh are the incense and essential oils used for the benefit of this chakra.

A healthy Throat Chakra allows us the ability to express ourselves and communicate effectively. An unhealthy Throat Chakra will cause us to feel invalidated and unheard. Artists must be cautious because if this chakra is unhealthy, it will block your creativity. A healthy Throat Chakra does not only affect how we express ourselves, it also affects how we hear others. This is essential to nurturing healthy relationships.

"WORDS HAVE POWER, CHOOSE YOURS WISELY." CAROL LYNNE SMITH.

Be careful what words you speak. In the beginning of the world, God spoke the world into existence. We have the same power. Life and death are in the power of the tongue. You can change your whole life based solely on the words you allow out of your mouth and into your ears.

During the time of my healing, I began doing something I had not thought to do before. I began to write out positive affirmations, words and love notes, and post them around my bedroom. I have notes on my mirror, taped to my dresser drawers, my walls and my bedroom door. I am surrounded by positive words and images. It does not take long for these words to become a part of who you are. During this stage of your journey, I encourage you to do the same. Use colorful note cards or index cards; whatever paper you wish but do it! I cannot express enough how beneficial this is.

In addition to writing these notes to yourself, I want you to send love notes to others. Think of a special person in your life; maybe you have a group of core friends you associate with, express yourself to them. Send them a letter, a text message or an email. Go on social media and post a sweet message to them. Use your sweet words of expression to tell them how amazing you think they are. The more you use your words to lift another person, the more powerful your Throat Chakra will become. So often we wait until they can no longer hear before we express how much we felt.

Affirmations:
"I speak with love and authority."
"I express myself lovingly and freely."
"What I have to say is worth listening to."

Reflection

Today would be a wonderful day to call up a friend and tell them just how much you adore them. In detail, tell them all the amazing qualities they have that you appreciate.

The more we use our voice for good, the more powerful it becomes.

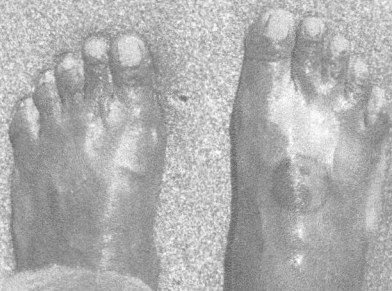

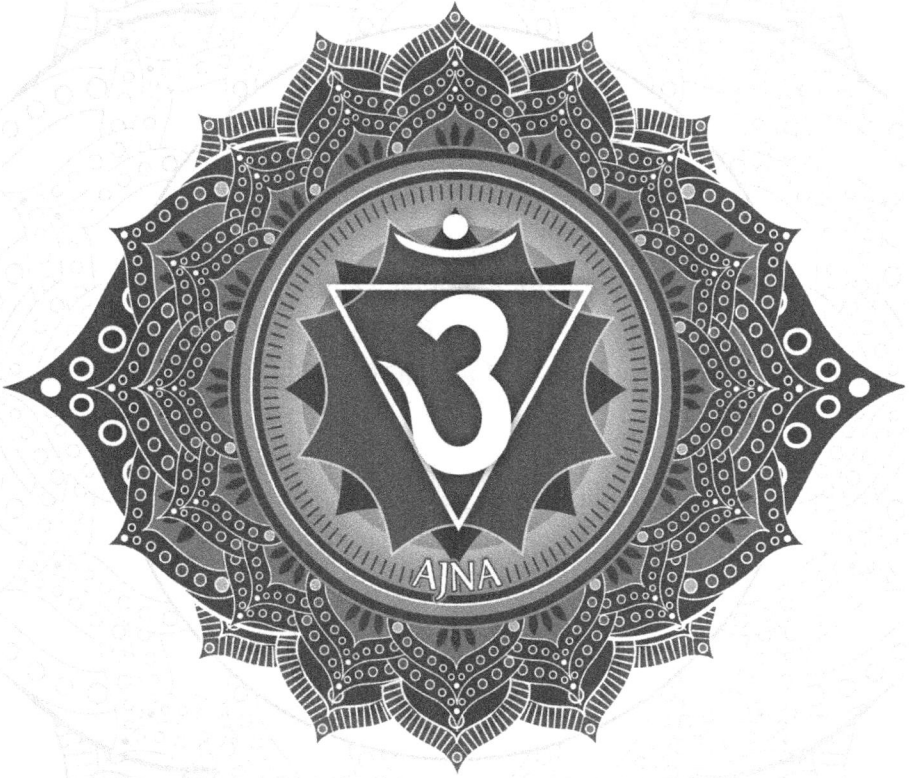

Chapter 18

Seeing is Believing

"During the darkest indigo midnight, yet will countless stars blossom."
Dr. SunWolf, Author

Although it is named the Third Eye Chakra, it is in fact the sixth chakra. The Sanskrit name is Ajna and it means "to perceive" or "to know." The location of the Third Eye Chakra is found directly between and slightly above our eyebrows. Its element is light, and its associative color is Indigo. It is symbolized by a lotus flower with two large petals on either side of it. The foods associated with a healthy sixth chakra include eggplant, blueberries, blackberries, as well as foods rich in Omega-3 such as salmon and chia seeds. The crystals used for balancing and healing this chakra include amethyst, fluorite, azurite and calcite; and the incense and essential oils are Rose geranium and hyacinth.

The Third Eye Chakra is at the core of our emotional intelligence and our ability to see beyond the obvious. A healthy Third Eye allows us to perceive things intuitively and increases our spiritual wisdom. An unhealthy Third Eye Chakra can cause headaches, neurological issues and learning disabilities. The Third Eye Chakra is often referred to as the Sixth Sense.

The meditation pose I use for the Third Eye Chakra is quite different than the others we have been using.

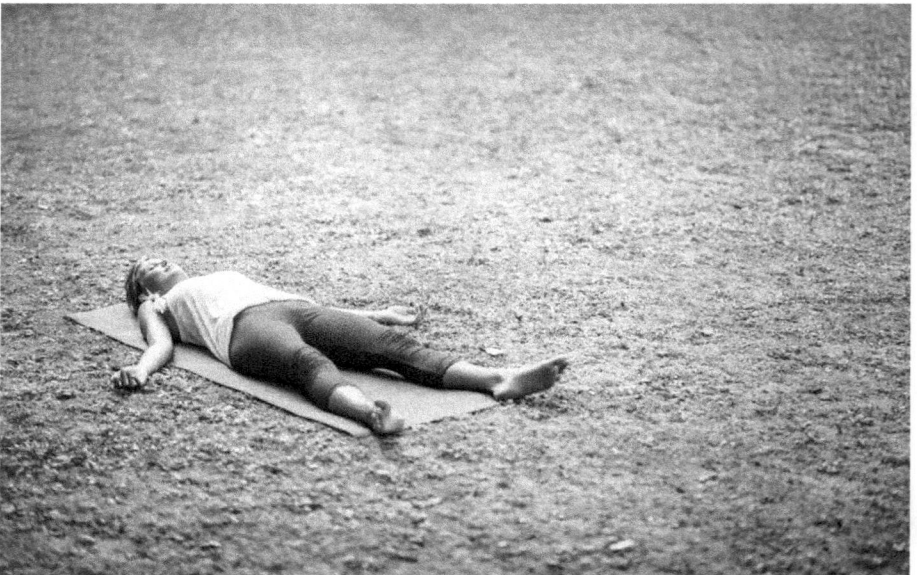

Find a comfortable place to lay down. This can be your bed, sofa or floor; anywhere that is comfortable and allows you a little privacy. Laying down on your back, place your chosen crystal on your Third Eye, keeping in mind this is between your eyebrows and then up a little. Human eyes should be closed, and your hands are facing upwards, and open making you available to receive all the knowledge the Universe is looking to give you.

Affirmations:
"I am full of wisdom."
"I am intuitive and powerful."
"I trust my inner voice, it is my teacher and my guide."

Reflection

When God gives you a vision and a purpose, He prepares you for it. However, you need to show up and make yourself available for it. If you are on a mission and ill-prepared for it, ask yourself if God purposed it.

This is why it is important to have a healthy Third Eye. It is essential on this journey that we are tuned in to the voice of God. We must spend time with Him, so that we might know Him and know His voice. Every time I reflect on this, I think back to Elijah and details of an event from the biblical book of First Kings 19.

The LORD said, "Go out and stand on the mountain in the presence of the LORD, for the LORD is about to pass by."

Then a great and powerful wind tore the mountains apart and shattered the rocks before the LORD, but the LORD was not in the wind. After the wind there was an earthquake, but the LORD was not in the earthquake. After the earthquake came a fire, but the LORD was not in the fire. And after the fire came a gentle whisper. When Elijah heard it, he pulled his cloak over his face and went out and stood at the mouth of the cave. (First Kings 19: 11-13 NIV)

All these powerful things happened, but because Elijah was familiar with God, he knew it was not Him. He was tuned in to God and therefore, when Elijah heard that gentle whisper, he approached, and it was then that God spoke to him.

A healthy Third Eye Chakra and a heart open to God, allows us to know Him, know His voice and act accordingly.

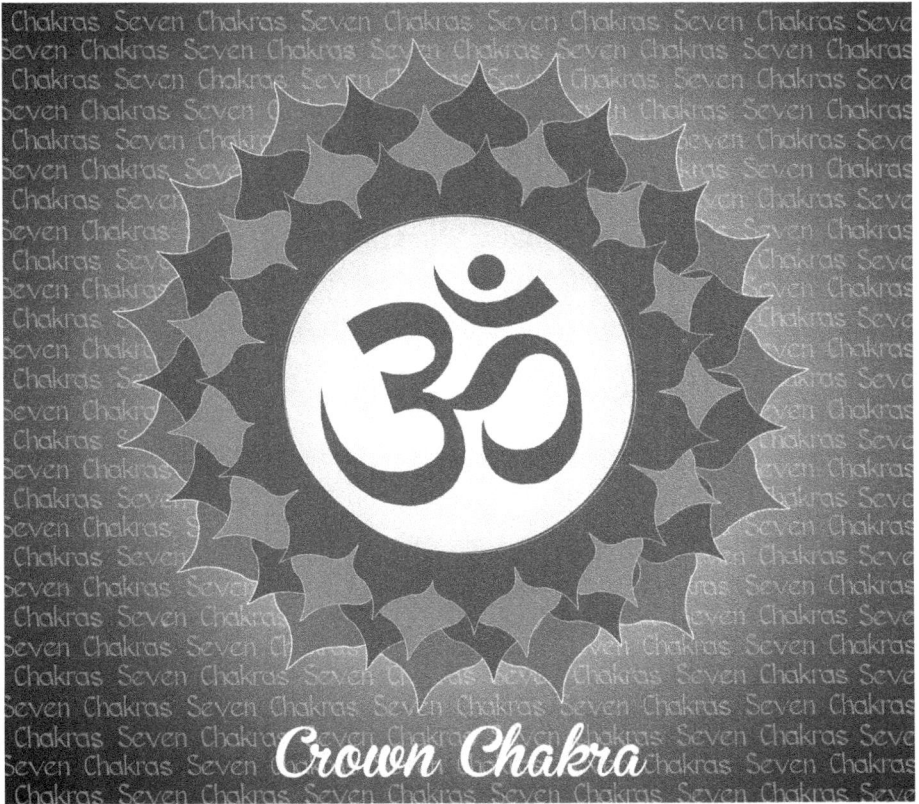

Crown Chakra

Chapter 19

---※---

Straighten Up Your Crown, Queen

"I think it pisses God off if we walk by the color purple in a field somewhere and don't notice it." Alice Walker, American novelist, The Color Purple

The seventh and final chakra is the Crown Chakra. The Sanskrit name for this chakra is Sahasrara which means "thousand petals." The lotus that symbolizes the Crown Chakra is the thousand-petalled flower. The Crown Chakra is located at the very top of our head and it is our connection with God and the Universe. The crystals associated with this chakra include Clear Quartz, Amethyst, White Jade, Diamonds and White tourmaline. The incense and essential oils are lavender and frankincense. The elements associated with the Crown Chakra are thought and universal energy, which is the vital energy for all living things. The color - purple.

There are no foods associated with this chakra and fasting is encouraged for a period while focusing on balancing and healing in this area. I highly recommend that you do not practice fasting unless you have been cleared to do so by your physician.

Having a healthy Crown Chakra is essential to this journey of wellness and wholeness. This is our connection to our Source; our connection to our spirituality. Having a healthy Crown Chakra allows us to be better human beings; selfless and knowledgeable.

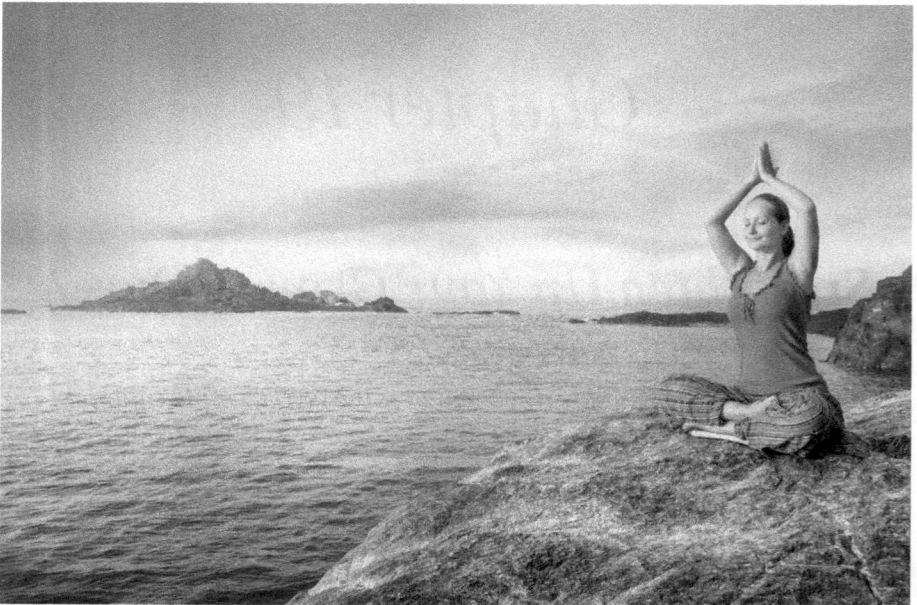

Meditating for the purposes of balancing and healing the Crown Chakra looks different than all the others. Although you are sitting in the Sukhasana pose, your hands should be raised above your head. Your chosen crystal should be able to sit on the top of your head. If for some reason you are not comfortable in this position, resume your traditional pose with your crystals in the palm of your hands.

Affirmations:
"I am tuned in to my higher power."
"I am connected to the Universe."
"I am connected and committed to God."

Reflection

I must admit, there are times when I wish things would come to me, as effortlessly as they seem to come to others. Then I am reminded that the struggle, is where I gain my strength.

In this moment, I understand that it is the struggle to escape the cocoon, that strengthens the wings of the butterfly.

The same is true for this journey to wellness and wholeness. There are moments that will test our resolve; we must push forward. We must not grow weary; we must stand strong. If you should fall, and you most certainly will, no need to worry. A temporary setback only becomes permanent if you allow it. Get up, dust yourself off, adjust your crown and pick up where you left off at.

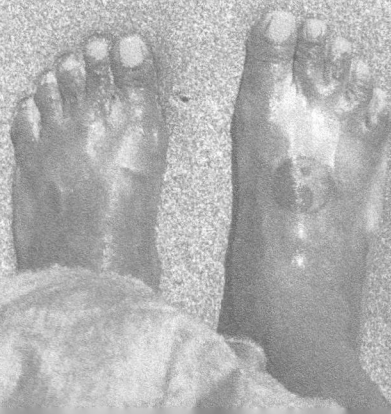

A healthy and freely flowing chi is essential to our journey to wellness and wholeness. Healthy and balanced chakras are essential to getting that energy flowing within us. Chakra health is the foundation of our healing, but we still have further to go. As we move further along into our journey, we will address more avenues of healing and supporting a healthy lifestyle.

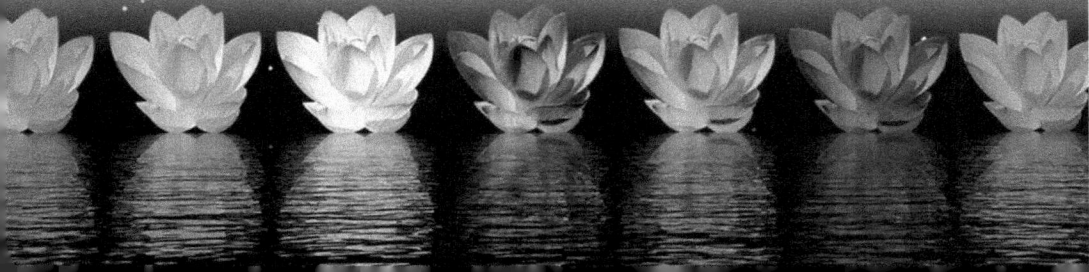

THE JOURNEY TO SELF

Chapter 20

———— ✳ ————

No New Thing Under the Sun

Chakra healing, crystals and essential oils as a pathway to womb healing are often categorized as "new age." There is nothing new about these methods of healing. New age is a term used for alternative methods of healing that made their way to Western culture in the 1970s, but the practices themselves are quite ancient and these methods of healing existed long before modern-day synthetic medications.

"...there is nothing new under the sun" (Ecclesiastes 1:9, NIV).

Womb healing is also not new. In fact, I would argue that Jesus Himself was the first to do so. In the biblical Gospels of Mark and Luke, we read of a woman who had an issue of blood for twelve years. The Bible tells us that she had seen many physicians, but none could cure her. She had heard that Jesus was nearby and by faith she knew that if she could get close enough to Him to just touch His clothing, just the energy from His clothing alone would be enough to heal her.

This issue of blood (as it is called in the Bible), is not about a woman bleeding for twelve years from her finger, her lip or her ear – it is about a woman bleeding from her vaginal cavity and the source of that bleeding began in her womb. When this woman touched the clothes that Jesus was wearing, the energetic power was so strong that Jesus noticed it. He asked those around Him to identify the source. They were unable to because the crowd was so thick. The woman who was immediately healed made herself known to Jesus. In Mark 5: 34, Jesus turned to the woman and said, "Daughter, your faith has healed you. Go in peace and be freed from your suffering" (NIV). What we see here is womb healing.

God wants us healed and He wants us whole. He has gifted us with so many avenues of healing, but we must be open to them. Many women have waited in vain to be whole again, while the pathway to wholeness was within their reach – had they only extended that reach outside of the box they (and society) had created for them.

Chapter 21

Let's Go to the Moon, Baby!

Looking back over the last 30-plus years of my life, I cannot help but regret how much time I wasted feeling doomed as I stared at a calendar seeing the dark days approaching. The dark days; that seven-day period where women feel as if the world has come to a stand-still because we are experiencing our moon cycles.

The moon cycle can be a difficult and painful experience for women who have fibroid tumors, endometriosis and other difficulties with the reproductive organs. It is essential that we get medical treatment for these abnormalities.

Except for a medical condition, the moon cycle should be a beautiful experience for a woman. During ancient times, a woman was honored during her bleeding cycles. Menstrual blood was used to nourish crops and men added it to their red wine believing that it would elevate their spiritual knowledge and power. Having a menstrual cycle was an honor amongst Goddesses.

Thousands of years later, our society shifted and a woman experiencing her moon cycle was looked upon as dirty. That stigma still haunts us today. We have the power to change that; not for the world at large, but certainly our little world. The moon cycle is physical proof that your body is still functioning and has the power to renew itself. This is a time of shedding and rejuvenation.

Rituals are important to healing the womb. Creating your own monthly rituals will allow you to embrace this time as the gift it truly is. This is a time of shedding what does not become us and embracing what is to come.

On the first day of your moon cycle, write out your intentions for the month. Monthly goals should be reasonable as you only have about 28 days to accomplish them. Try choosing a room, or space in your home that needs your attention and focus on clearing that space this month. Does your bookshelf still house children's books that your kids have outgrown? Does your closet need to be organized? Set a goal for clearing these spaces.

This is also an exciting time to focus on what you are eating. Replace your porkchops with an extra side of green vegetables. Your body is going through a period of natural cleansing and you can aid in this process by eating foods that are medicinal. Drink lots of warm tea. Abdominal cramps during your moon cycle is caused by blood clotting. Warm beverages promote a healthy blood flow. There are several teas available on the market for supporting a healthy cycle. I am partial towards the "Woman's Moon Cycle" tea by Yogi. All teas are created equally, but Yogi adds an inspirational message to each one of their tea bags and as we learned earlier, it is essential that we surround ourselves with positive words.

Meditating and grounding are necessary during your moon cycle. I love the rain and I enjoy walking barefoot on wet grass. However, I do not recommend that you do that during this time. If you are going to do some grounding during your moon cycle, do so when the ground is dry. Your body is more open during this time and we must be protective of it. When meditating during this period, find a position that is comfortable for you. This can be laying comfortable on your back; or sitting in the Sukhasana pose.

Your choice of crystals is important during this time. The Moonstone crystal is highly recommended as you go through this period of shedding and renewal. The moonstone crystal is associated with the goddess. It is a symbol of fertility and sensuality, feminine empowerment and healing. Meditating with the moonstone allows you to connect with the sacred feminine and embrace her.

The moon cycle is not a time of mourning, it is a time of honoring yourself and other goddesses. This is not a time of hiding out at home for seven days, it is time of rejoicing, singing and dancing. Your body is healthy, your spirit is cleansing, and your mind is renewing. Your chi is flowing, your wheels are spinning; you are sacred, healthy and whole.

Reflection

Today feels like a great day to remind you how beautiful you are. You are an amazing woman, perfectly crafted by God. Your body is not only His temple, it is His greatest creation. Take some time rejoicing in that truth.

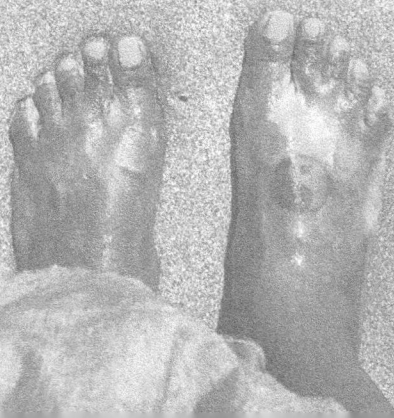

Chapter 22

---✳---

Making Peace with Your Scar

"The wound is the place where the light enters you." Rumi, Poet

As I began to physically heal from my hysterectomy, it became obvious that the scar that remained was not diminishing as I had hoped. Every time I look at a mirror, there it is staring back at me. A three-dimensional reminder of the physical trauma that had taken place there. After months of stressing over my scar, it was obvious to me that it was not going anywhere, and I needed to make peace with it.

"...and I said to my body softly – I want to be your friend – it took a long breath and replied – I have been waiting my whole life for this." Nayyirah Waheed, Poet

Making peace with my surgical scar was not as easy as I had hoped it would be. In addition to the physical appearance, it was irritating. There were times when the itching was unbearable. I knew the benefits of essential oils; so, when it came time for me to look at ways of tending to my scar, that is where I started. Frankincense and myrrh, as it turned out, weren't simply great gifts for the little baby Jesus, they were also great medicinal oils for my wound.

Frankincense is easy to work with when creating a healing oil or salve, but myrrh is a little trickier. Myrrh is sappy and it needs a little heating for it to become pliable. Using sunflower oil (or an oil of your choosing such as jojoba, olive or coconut) as a carrier/base oil, prepare an ointment using frankincense and myrrh. I want to remind you that carrier oils are necessary because essential oils can act as an irritant when placed directly on our skin. You can use 12 drops of essential oils for every fluid ounce of your carrier oils. You can also add some other fragrant essential oils to the mix. Lavender and geranium are delightfully scented, and they are essential to healing the sacred feminine. Another essential oil that is both fragrant and inexpensive is lemongrass oil. I would apply this mixture of oils to my scar about twice a day, and after about a month, the itching eased, and I made peace with my scar.

WRITE IT OUT

Not all our scars are physical. The trauma from toxic relationships, physical abuse and chronic illness can leave emotional scars. Journaling is an effective way of working through the process of healing our emotional scar tissue. Journaling has many benefits and is an effective tool on our journey to wellness and wholeness. Journaling can boost our moods and it is a tool recommended by health practitioners for people dealing with PTSD. Journaling is cathartic and allows our creative juices to flow. It is an effective means of tackling depression and anxiety, and it allows us to express ourselves in an environment that is safe.

Journaling gives us the means for making peace with our brokenness.

Reflection

Scars are a sign that some healing has taken place. Emotional scars mean the same thing. Scars are proof that you survived. You are not a victim of your experiences, you are a conqueror, an overcomer, a survivor!

Goddess, you got this!

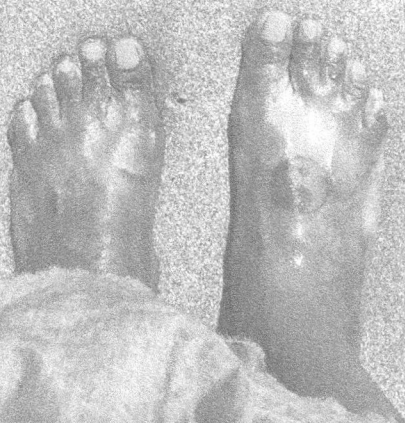

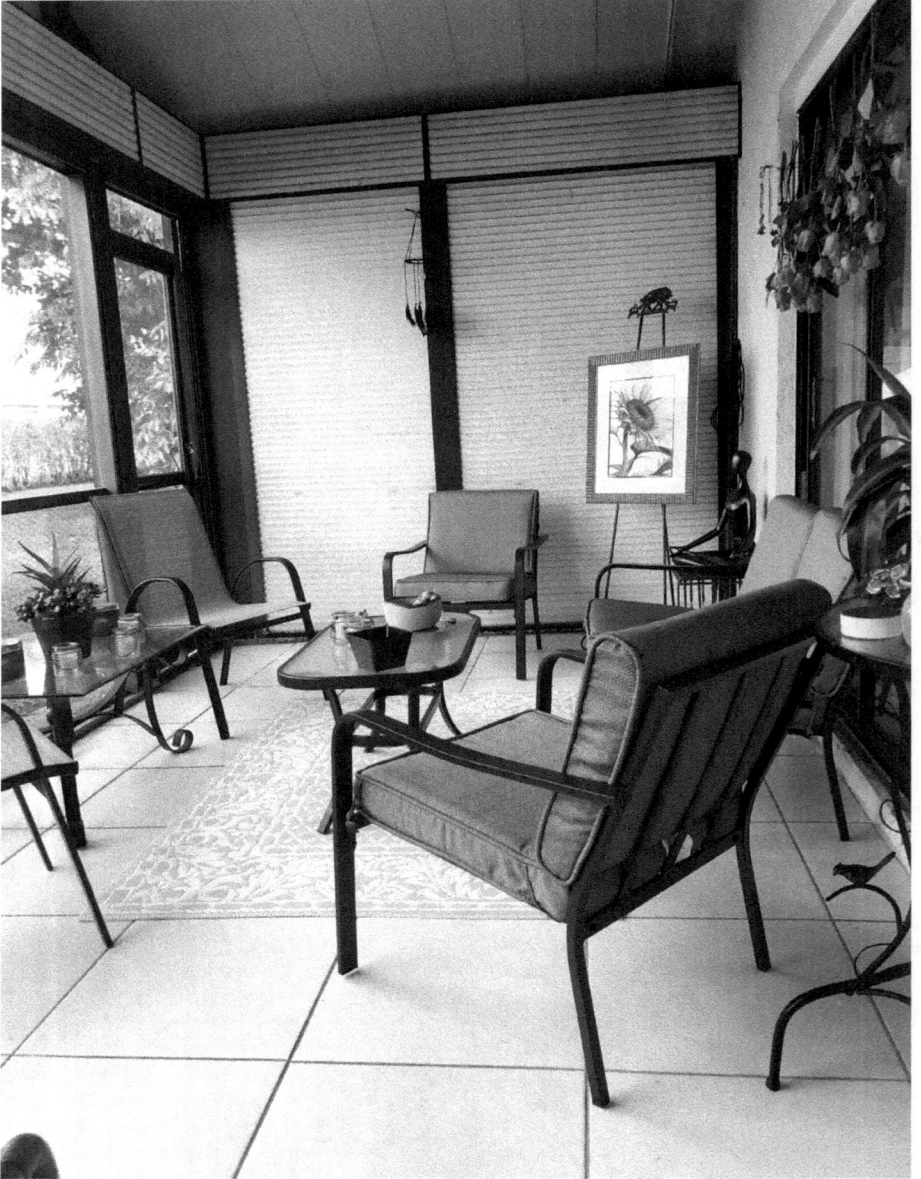

Chapter 23

Hey! That's My Spot!

Archie Bunker, Martin Crane, Sheldon Cooper; aside from all being fictional television characters, they each have another thing in common. They each have their own spot, and you better not dare sit in it. Guess what? It's time you have your own spot; your own sacred space. This is a place that belongs only to you. It can be a chair, or a whole room. Maybe it's just a small corner in a larger room. No matter how large or small the space is, it needs to be yours, and yours alone.

Every woman needs a sanctuary; a place where her spirit can take a break and relax. We spend so much time catering to the needs of others, we need a place to refuel.

Obviously, how you use the space will be determined by the type of space it is. If your home only allows for you to have a sacred chair, place a beautiful throw pillow there and let that be the space you read in, and drink your lavender tea. If your space is a small corner in a larger room, perhaps that is the space you meditate in as well. If you are fortunate enough to have a larger space to call your own, the possibilities can be endless. If you have a shed in your backyard filled with junk, clean it out and turn it into a she shed! Choose your sacred spot, then make it yours.

THE SUN GODDESS CAFÉ

I turned my patio into my sacred space. I decorated it with cute outdoor furniture, plants and decorative items and named it: The Sun Goddess Café. Most mornings and evenings I find myself in the café saying my prayers, drinking my coffee or tea, reading a book or journaling, meditating or having a conversation with a friend. Shortly after designing the space, I opened it up as a gathering place for other women. I use this space to teach other women how to heal through conversations, workshops, energy clearing and chakra readings. Although this is indeed my sacred space, opening it up and allowing other women to gather and heal makes the space more sacred.

Chapter 24

———※———

Holy Smoke!

The journey to wellness and wholeness is as much about our physical environment as it is internal. To support good health, we must create an environment that is conducive to such.

Your home must become your sanctuary; your safe space. Do an inventory of your home. Is there something there that no longer suits the woman you are now? Perhaps there are items in your home that have negative attachments to them. They were given to you by an ex-partner, and that relationship was toxic. Sell it or give it away. Rid your space of it.

Your sanctuary should be filled with things that evoke a sense of joy, peace and happiness. If you love bright colors, fill your space with those colors regardless of the season. If you love earth tones, decorate your home with those colors, even if the season calls for yellow. Connect with your home, this is your sanctuary.

Once you have physically cleared the space, you are then tasked with clearing the energy that exists there. Sacred smoke is an amazing tool for doing this. The most common method for this is white sage, but Palo Santo also known as Holy Wood, is a beautifully fragrant alternative. Historically, Native Americans took part in smudging for the purpose of spiritually cleansing a person, or place. Smudging is the act of burning white sage, Palo Santo and even incense for the purpose of cleansing.

Smudging can be done at any time you feel it necessary, but there are times when I highly recommend it.

Before you begin your journey to wellness and wholeness, make sure to smudge your home. You are clearing out toxic energy and making room for the goddess being healed within you. When you have guests in your home, their energy comes with them, but it does not always leave when they leave. Smudge your home after your guests leave. If your home is like mine and it is a place where people gather, smudge before and after a gathering. Smudge your home after an argument with your partner; smudge you and your partner too. Smudge your home after you have recovered from a cold or another similar outbreak. It is also important to smudge a new home before you move into it.

It is important that you open your windows and doors as sage does get very smoky. Also be advised that the intense smoke is enough to set off your smoke detectors, so be careful not to place the burning herbs near them.

Smudging clears your space of all energy both negative and positive, so after you finish smudging, burn a fragrant incense or scented candle to invite the sweetness back in. Sweet grass is a beautiful herb to burn after smudging, but it can be awfully hard to find, and it does not hold a flame well.

Say your prayers and affirmations and allow the sacred smoke to take your words directly into the Universe.

USING SACRED SMOKE TO CLEANSE YOUR TEMPLE

Sage is as beneficial for your temple – your body, as it is for your home. You can spend time with a Shamanic healer and give them permission to cleanse you with sage, or you can easily cleanse yourself.

There is a space in my home that has a large bay window. I sit there on a stool or on the floor, I light the sage wand and using a crisscross style motion, I smudge myself from my Crown Chakra to my Root Chakra. I open my legs and allow the sacred smoke entry into my most sacred space. When I am done, I place the smoking sage in a safe dish, and allow it to burn out on its own.

Find a space in your sanctuary where you can comfortably sit and smudge yourself. A space with glass windows and doors that allow for natural light to come in would be ideal. Sit down, light your sage and wait for the flame to disappear; close your eyes and let the smoke from the sage find you.

Reflection

What a wonderful opportunity you have been gifted with. Your home is your sanctuary and it is designed to cater to the woman you are. Your home has been cleared of everything that no longer suits you and you have created an environment that is nurturing to you, everyone who lives there and everyone who crosses your threshold.

You are right where you are supposed to be, and your home is now a divine reflection of that.

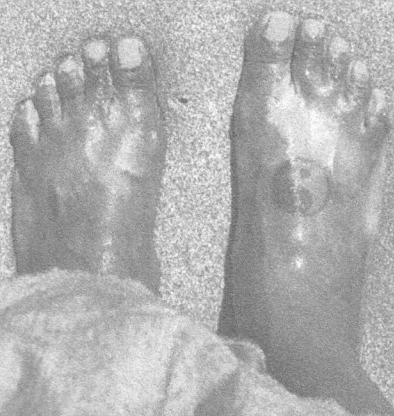

Chapter 25

---※---

The Key to Healing is to Never See Yourself Broken Beyond Repair

There were so many times on my journey where I felt like I was standing on the edge of a cliff. I thought for sure I would just give up and jump! Then God stepped in, turned on the lights and I realized that I was not on the edge of a cliff, I was on the edge of a breakthrough! The same is true with our healing. So often it can feel like it is not even worth the try; because we feel so far removed from the healthier version of ourselves. For me, it had been over thirty years of brokenness, and often it felt like it was too late for me to heal.

I was wrong. The key to my healing was to first understand that it was not too late. I had become complacent in my brokenness, but I was not broken beyond repair.

"Your wound is probably not your fault - but your healing is your responsibility." Shraddha Sreedev, Writer

The same truth exists inside of you. No matter how long you have been wounded, no matter how long you have been nursing a scar – you can still heal. It is easy to remain in the broken state because healing requires work, but it is worth it. In the biblical book of Joel, chapter 2 – there is a story of restoration. There we find God instructing us to repent for the years of brokenness and in return He offers restoration of all the time that was lost. I believe this translates over to our healing. When we begin the process of healing, we are rewarded with restoration. We can have a renewed sense of time and energy and can find ourselves in position to do things that we had only dreamed of prior to our healing.

I am not saying that this is an easy process. Healing takes time and dedication. We must put the work in! The closer you are to your breakthrough, the stronger the resistance you begin to feel. Push through it. You are worth the healing!

Reflection

What goals have you placed on the back burner because of your own brokenness? Allow yourself the opportunity to heal and free up that space to begin to carry out your goals. I speak from experience when I say that brand - new life awaits you!

Goddess, you got this!

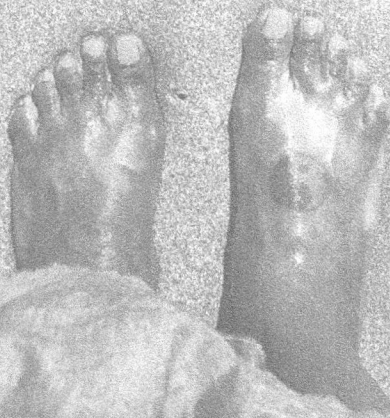

There are days when I stumble and fall while on this journey. I begin to believe that my work may have been in vain. Then I realize that I must stand back up, brush the dirt off my knees, bandage my wounded ego and start over from the point where I fell. I am never damaged beyond repair.

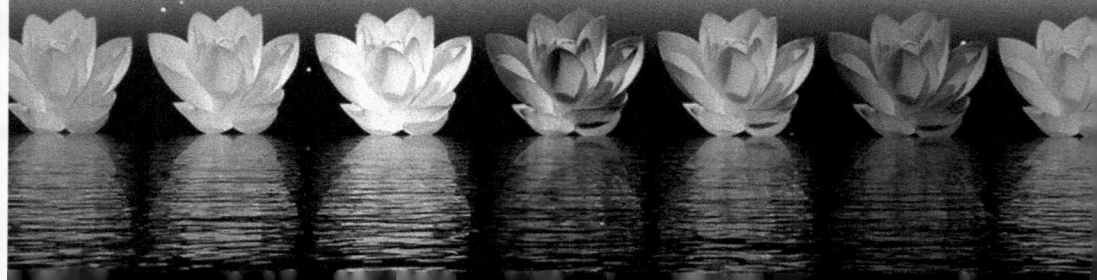

Chapter 26

※

Food for Your Spirit

I love going out for dinner. I sit down at the table, look over the menu and decide what I want to eat and drink. Before you know it, some kind soul is bringing hot food and a cold drink to my table. I pay for my meal and leave my dirty dishes on the table. This is the good life!

As much as I enjoy a meal I did not have to cook, there is something so refreshing about preparing my own healthy meals and drinks at home. When we began our discussion on chakras, I talked a little about juicing and how important it is along with the value of a green diet. I love the full process of cleaning my fruits and vegetables and preparing them for juicing and making smoothies, or for cooking a healthy meal. It does take time, but I have turned this into a ritual.

When I am cleaning and peeling beets, I meditate. I do the same when I am cleaning carrots, slicing apples or separating the kale leaves from the stem. I am aware that this food I am touching will be used for my nourishment, as well as for the benefit of my partner and my family. When I am prepping these healthy items, it feels like I am creating art. The colors of the beets, carrots and apples mixed; the kale being stir fried in the wok – ARTFUL!

Juicing and preparing vegetables for cooking does not need to be tedious. Invest in a juicer with a larger mouth which will cut down on your prep time. Play inspirational music in the kitchen and turn this space into a sanctuary. Smile, dance and sing while you cook and allow that good energy to absorb into your food, which will in turn go back into your body.

Practicing this type of mindful cooking will not only make your food taste better, I believe it increases the nutritional benefits. No matter what, you will enjoy this part of your journey.

Reflection

I challenge you this week to commit to cooking your meals at home. For the next seven days only eat meals that you have lovingly prepared for yourself. Turn your kitchen into a sanctuary and allow your food to be a form of artistic expression. At the end of the week, take some time to reflect on how you felt while preparing and eating your meals.

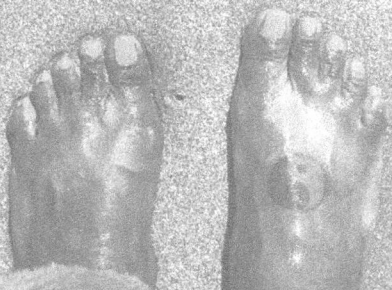

Chapter 27

---·※·---

Clarity Comes

During my period of brokenness, I allowed so much toxicity. I made room for things in my life that I otherwise would not have. I found it difficult to say no to things that did not suit me. I wasted time and energy on temporary situations, relationships and people. I had so much regret over the years, that I became sick when healthy was an available possibility.

HEALING BROUGHT ME CLARITY

After I was well on my journey to wellness and wholeness, I created a pathway that would allow me to help other women to heal. Through workshops, one-on-one meetings and through my writings, I have attracted a tribe of goddesses, intent on healing. Taking the time to teach other women how to heal from their own brokenness has been rewarding. I have discovered that the more I help others heal, the more I am healed. The relationship between a healer and the person being healed is reciprocal.

As you find your own way from brokenness to wellness and wholeness, be sure to bring other women along with you. Create your own tribe; be the light that lights the path for other women. Heal by healing others.

You will find many blessings on this journey.

Chapter 28

I Leave You with This

"When I arrived there, I saw a great number of trees on each side of the river." Then He said to me, "This water flows toward the eastern region and goes down into the Arabah, where it enters the Dead Sea. When it empties into the sea, the salty water there becomes fresh." "Swarms of living creatures will live wherever the river flows. There will be large numbers of fish, because this water flows there and makes the salt water fresh; so, where the river flows everything will live."
(Ezekiel 47:7-9, NIV)

As you continue your journey:
- Speak your own truth; do not allow others to tell your story, they are sure to get some details wrong.
- Strengthen your intellectual muscles; there is always learning to be done.
- Release bitterness otherwise it will leave a bad taste in your mouth.
- Continue to experience love, even if you have been hurt before.
- Nourish healthy relationships.
- Eat healthy foods, you only get this one body.
- Focus on yourself, do not neglect yourself for the comfort of others.
- Commune with nature – at least once a week commit to spending time outdoors.
- Remain connected to the Earth below you, and the Heaven above you.

- Remain in awe of the Sun and the Moon.
- Embrace each moment.
- Honor yourself – honor your body. Not everyone is eligible to spend time in your Yoniverse.
- Commune with God; and may everything that flows from your sacred temple bring life and renewal to everything it touches – the same way the river that flowed from the temple in the biblical book of Ezekiel gave life and made fresh everything it touched.

...And remember, the Universe is conspiring to give you everything you need.

We are on this journey together. We all have comparable stories and experiences (with a few variations).

There are times when you will need to share your story or your journey with other women. In sharing your story, they may begin to find themselves and their need for healing. Transparency on this journey is essential to your healing and to the healing of those around you.

The light from your flame is not diminished by lighting the candle of the woman next to you.

Goddess, you got this!

Chapter 29

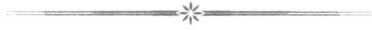

The Goddess Soul Contract

Now that you have read this book, the real work begins. Go back through each chapter and apply the principles and practices to your life and to your healing. Below, you will find the Goddess Soul Contract. This is the contract that you will make with yourself knowing that every other woman who reads this book will be making the same declaration of healing. We are placing that vibrational energy out into the Universe and collectively healing!

Here we go!

GODDESS SOUL CONTRACT

I accept who I am right now, while I continue to make room for my growth.

I am in renewal – both my mind, my body and my spirit.

I release myself from the sins of my past. I forgive myself for self-inflicted hurts, and I forgive others for the hurt they caused me. I forgive myself for the hurt I caused others.

I will show up every day for the woman I see reflected in the mirror.

I will love her by giving thought as to what I wear, I drink, I eat, and I think.

I embrace me, I accept me, I love me.

I honor the goddess that is me.

And so - it is.

I HAVE SO MANY QUESTIONS!

Q. How do you burn white sage for smudging, clearing and cleansing?

A. I like to use a long lighter, one like you would use to light a candle or charcoal on a grill. Let the sage get a good little fire going so that it will emit a great amount of smoke. One you see a nice amount of smoke, extinguish the flame. Please note that the fire will at times extinguish itself. This is fine.

Q. What is a safe dish to use to set your lit or smoking sage in?

A. There are many safe dishes available for purchase, however, there is probably something in your kitchen you can use. You can use a microwave safe dish; you should line the dish with sand or soil to ensure that it is safe from breaking. You can also use a soap stone dish, an abalone shell or a cast iron dish. These can all be bought online or found in metaphysical stores.

Q. Is it safe to wash my crystal gemstones?

A. Most crystals can be washed, however there are a few that can be damaged or dissolved by water. Please do a simple internet search to see if the stones you bought can be washed.

Q. How do I clear the energy from my crystals?

A. There a couple of methods used. Some place their crystals under the New Moon (the period when the Moon is not illuminated), or under the Full Moon (the period when the Moon is fully illuminated). You can do an internet search of Moon Cycles to find out when the next New or Full Moon is occurring. The method I most commonly use is sage. I light my sage and allow the smoke to surround my crystals. I meditate and speak my intentions for my stones. There are also some crystals that clear other crystals. Selenite for example is a great clearing crystal. You can place your stones on top of selenite, and within a few minutes they will be clear. Please note that some stones – selenite being one of them - do not need to be cleared. Again, do a little research on your new gemstones to find out which ones require clearing and which ones do not.

Q. Can I use the method of healing you have written about instead of going to a doctor?

A. Absolutely NOT! The methods I use are for the purpose of emotional and spiritual healing. These methods worked because they went with the consult and treatment of my doctors and surgeons, whose care I looked for first. It was not until after my physical healing from surgery was complete that I began to apply these methods. Energy healing is not a substitute for physical healing. Physical healing needs care from board certified physicians.

Q. Can I be a woman of God and use these methods of healing?

A. Absolutely! Energy and vibrational healing are not a religious. This type of healing is not a replacement for God; it is another avenue God uses to bring healing. It is a practical way in which we can take responsibility for our own health and well-being.

Q. Carol, what are your thoughts on yoni steams, yoni pearls and the other products that are being marketed for vaginal insertion?

A. Beyond the yoni egg, I am not a proponent for anything that gets inserted into the Yoni. As far as the steam choice goes, I believe the goddess bath is a safer one. Of course, you should speak with your board-certified OB/GYN before using any products of this nature.